D0630777

MERCY AND MADNESS

Dr. Mary Archard Latham's Tragic Fall from Female Physician to Felon

BEVERLY LIONBERGER HODGINS

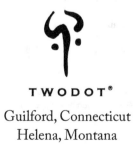

TWODOT®

Guilford, Connecticut
Helena, Montana

A · TWODOT® · BOOK

An imprint of Globe Pequot, the trade division of
The Rowman & Littlefield Publishing Group, Inc.
4501 Forbes Blvd., Ste. 200
Lanham, MD 20706
www.rowman.com

Distributed by NATIONAL BOOK NETWORK

Copyright © 2022 by Beverly Lionberger Hodgins

All rights reserved. No part of this book may be reproduced in any form or by any electronic or mechanical means, including information storage and retrieval systems, without written permission from the publisher, except by a reviewer who may quote passages in a review.

British Library Cataloguing in Publication Information available

Library of Congress Cataloging-in-Publication Data available

ISBN 978-1-4930-5974-4 (cloth : alk. paper)
ISBN 978-1-4930-5975-1 (electronic)

♾️™ The paper used in this publication meets the minimum requirements of American National Standard for Information Sciences—Permanence of Paper for Printed Library Materials, ANSI/ NISO Z39.48-1992.

To my mother,
Roberta Elaine Witcraft Lionberger,
whose love of books and research
was the light illuminating my path
and
to my grandmother,
Charity Idora Archerd Witcraft

CONTENTS

INTRODUCTION

The narrative of young Mary Archard from Ohio could have unfolded as follows: Farm girl makes good. Marries well. Breaks barriers, becoming a physician in the late 1800s. Journeys west without her husband to improve her health. Establishes her practice as a specialist in diseases of women and children. Lives and works for twenty-nine years while watching Spokane Falls, Washington Territory, successively burn, rebuild, and grow into the bustling city of Spokane, Washington State.

Inside her office in the city—as Dr. Mary A. Latham—and inside both homes and hospitals, her patients are women, children, *and* men who live in shacks below in Poverty Flats and above in the mansions of Browne's Addition belonging to empire builders and silver mine owners, and in every type of place in between. Her exceptional skills are needed for everything from setting broken bones to delivering babies—perhaps her favorite task—to performing surgery. With each passing year, she gains a stronger, more brilliant and diverse reputation: extraordinary physician, generous philanthropist, outspoken writer, defender of unfortunate girls and abandoned infants, and devoted mother.

The combination of Mary's love of travel and her curious intellect takes her south to California and into the country of Mexico, back to Ohio, and likely east to New York City. From San Francisco she boards a steamer ship to Alaska, becoming the first woman from Washington State to travel to the source of the Yukon River. She dreams of seeing Paris and the Panama Canal.

The best, perhaps most predictable version of magnanimous Mary's saga would document her continuing along this beneficent and oft-inspiring path of service before retiring to enjoy old age at her ranch near Long Lake in Spokane County, Washington.

But the best version of her story would not be the true version.

Through five decades Mary lived an extraordinary and satisfying life. However, in 1903, her path would meet a switchback of enormous proportions, with Mary suffering dearly after the devastating loss of a son. Some would say she also lost her mind. Records exist of opinions expressed by both physicians and friends who believed that following the death of her son, Mary suffered from both depression and dementia, along with the aftereffects of a stroke. Yet, these opinions would be disregarded by powerful men when Mary needed them most.

During Mary's early years in Spokane Falls, she made several shrewd real estate purchases, buying numerous city lots and acreage, where she planted orchards and harvested many varieties of fruit. The volume of her property holdings identified her as a wealthy woman.

In collaboration with another female physician, Mary opened a women's maternity hospital in downtown Spokane in 1892, proudly listing it in the city directory. The achievement of a long-held goal for Mary, there is curiously no mention of it in the following year's directory. It's possible the property was lost during the financial Panic of 1893, when many banks and lending institutions were forced to call in mortgage loans. By the time Mary had opened the hospital, she was separated from her husband of twenty-five years, Dr. Edward H. Latham. Latham went north to serve as government physician to the tribes on the Colville Indian Reservation.

Despite this marital setback, Mary achieved a wealth of influence inside the city by variously serving as president, vice president, secretary, and treasurer for a number of organizations and associations, including the Humane Society, the Spokane Sorosis Club, the Home of the Friendless, the Union Library Association, the Horticultural Society—formerly the all-male Fruit Growers Association—and the Queen Isabella Association.

At one time, Mary was sworn in as a deputy sheriff, becoming the first woman ever deputized in the State of Washington.

From her earliest years in Ohio through her first fifteen years in Spokane, it became apparent that Mary's accomplishments were the product of a remarkable mind and an indomitable will. In Spokane, she was not afraid to associate with accomplished men, including performing surgery in tandem with a male physician—and it was not her husband. Everyone knew Mary. But everyone did not have her best interests at heart. It began to appear—as Mary's expanding vulnerabilities became manifest—that some, even some whom she considered friends, were all too eager to take advantage of the well-to-do Mary.

After the death of her son—that trauma being compounded by the stroke—Mary began making unwise and, some would accuse, nefarious financial decisions. She would fall under the influence of men who attempted to profit from their acquaintance with her, perhaps driven by that age-old sin, *envy*.

During her fifth decade, she was surrounded by professional men. Some who had respected her now mocked her as she began to face lawsuits and finally, a more-than-weeklong trial inside the Superior Court of Spokane County in 1905, where she was circumstantially convicted of arson by a jury of twelve men. Mary would lose more than her freedom in the following years, as creditors would come calling and land holdings disappear.

What appears to be the beginning of the end for Mary occurs in January of 1906, when, at the age of sixty-one, in frail health and with a pronounced limp, Mary is escorted through the doors of the Washington State Penitentiary to serve her four-year sentence at hard labor. Even then, Mary does not give up, continuing to write letters to prison officials regarding parole, and later, a pardon.

But it is not prison life that kills Mary; it is her soft heart and never-ending willingness to administer care to those in need. She was the epitome of J. L. Rockey's description of a dedicated physician in the book, *History of Clermont County, Ohio.* "The true physician is not only ever ready to obey the calls of the sick, but his mind is thoroughly imbued with the greatness of his mission and the deep responsibility he habitually incurs in its discharge."

Retired from official practice, Mary, "ever ready to obey the calls of the sick," was moved to care for a newborn, whom she had certainly delivered, suffering with pneumonia. Aged and frail, the vulnerable Mary contracts the disease. Later, her grandson and his mother hold vigil at her bedside. Mary dies on January 20, 1917, inside the Sacred Heart Hospital, where she once walked the halls dispensing health care, boundless goodwill, and compassion to her beloved patients in Spokane.

CHAPTER I

The Farmer's Five Daughters

One morning when I was a little girl of 4 I was sent by my mother to the barn to get eggs for breakfast [from] the manger . . .

I climbed up . . . and looking down . . . in the nest were not eggs indeed, but my little playmate Frisk, and with her, filling the nest to overflowing, were six little baby Frisks of all colors and as soft as silk.

Frisk looked up at me, wagged her tail, her eyes beaming with mother love and pride, as she cuddled her little ones closer to her.

Climbing down . . . with Frisk following close at my heels, and my apron full of little dogs, I ran home. . . .

My father stormed, was angry because the eggs which were to make his breakfast were not ready for him, and picking up the little, sprawling things, he, in the twinkling of an eye, settled the question of the "survival of the fittest" by dashing four of the six cruelly against the hard floor. The remaining two were put in a box and were not to be touched by anyone, and my father's law in that household was like the law of the Medes and Persians. . . .

Early in the morning I sought out my old playmate and found Frisk in her box, and with her the two little ones . . .

As I grew older, and heard my father in his prayer uttered thrice daily say, "Forgive our many sins," I felt sure there was one sin for which he could never be forgiven. . . .

One thing I remember most of all is, as I gazed into the nest where my mother had told me that [I] would find some little chickens, how

great my amazement was that I should find the puppies instead, and
wondered what life was and how it came.
    —*MARY A. LATHAM, "Stories of Canines,"*
    the Spokane Review, July 2, 1891

Mary Archard was the daughter of James and Jane Archard and grand-daughter of John Archerd, who arrived from Somersetshire [later called Somerset], England, to help settle the village of New Richmond in Clermont County, Ohio. In his book *Archerd: Family History*, William F. Archerd states that John named Mary's father after a "like-minded Presbyterian," James Whillden.

James Whillden Archard and Jane Warren were "solemnized" in marriage on April 13, 1837, by George Beecher, according to Clermont County marriage records. George Beecher was an abolitionist Presbyterian minister from Batavia, Ohio, and the brother of Harriet Beecher Stowe, author of *Uncle Tom's Cabin*.

James and Jane built their home as described in a family letter, "perched on the top of the hill looking as if a little wind or a little push would send it tumbling down into the river." This was not far from the birthplace of future president Ulysses S. Grant.

Jane's birth is remembered as that of the first white child born in New Richmond. Her father, James Warren, built the first shingled log house and later purchased Ivy Brook Farm, where Jane was born. The Quaker ancestors of Jane's mother were said to have been "among those who struck the first axe in the forest primeval." Descended from early American immigrants, James and Jane were not intimidated by task or trial. Jane's long line of astounding female ancestors included the daughter of the founder of New Richmond, John Light.

<hr />

It's curious to find that within the pages of the last will and testament of James, his last name "Archard" was clearly spelled two ways: with an ending of *ard* and an ending of *erd*. The same is true of Jane. This use of alternate spellings occurred throughout their lives and the lives of their children. In order to eliminate confusion, and except for immigrant

John Archerd, the family's surname will be spelled *Archard* within this text.

It's been suggested the surname originated from the word, *orchard*. In *Archerd: Family History*, Mary's sister, Eliza, is quoted as saying: "There is little doubt but that the name was originally Orchard and was changed to Archard by the peculiar vernacular of their place of residence, Orchard becoming Archard just as horse became harse."

＿＿＿

Jane gave birth to five daughters and one son over a period of twelve years.

First born, on January 4, 1838, was Eliza Jane, whose education began at home until she was enrolled at the Clermont Academy, located in "a neat little hamlet on the Ohio River, two miles above New Richmond." A number of institutions were eager for Clermont Academy graduates, the academy being considered "a school of higher learning than the public schools can afford."

Eliza's name appears on the 1857 roll for Antioch College in Yellow Springs, Ohio, where she graduated in 1861. Eventually, Eliza accepted a position at the Indianapolis High School, where she went to teach German and Latin. There, "her refusal to accept lower wages than the male teachers received led to a reform in that matter which is still observed." In April of 1865, she resigned from her post as "head assistant in Franklin School," perhaps because her petition from two years earlier "asking for the salary of head assistant, was referred to the Auditing Committee,—a virtual refusal of the petition."

In the same year she resigned, Eliza took her expanding talent with the pen and became a regular contributor to the *Saturday Evening Post* of Philadelphia, under the pen name Zig.

In 1869, she married Dr. George Conner, who became a prominent physician with a "lucrative practice" in Cincinnati. They had one child in 1873, Halstead Archard Conner. As a contributor to the *Cincinnati Commercial* newspaper, Eliza was identified by her initials, E. A.

Eliza moved alone to New York City, probably around 1884, when she became the literary editor of the *New York World*, which had been purchased by Joseph Pulitzer. Pulitzer vowed to concentrate on human-interest stories, and to "expose all fraud and sham, fight all public evils and abuses and to battle for the people with earnest sincerity." This description seems to fit with the work of Eliza; and yet, she resigned from the paper in 1886.

Eliza may have resigned to focus her energy and passion on the suffrage movement. On June 22, 1894, in the *Joliet News* of Joliet, Illinois, Eliza's name is included in a noteworthy list: "No matter how the petitions are received by the constitutional convention, the present interest taken by the society women of New York is of itself a great victory for the pioneer like Mrs. Elizabeth Cady Stanton, Mrs. Lillie Devereux Blake, Mrs. Mary A. Livermore, Miss Susan B. Anthony and the host of younger women like Mrs. Eliza Archard Conner, Helen Gardener, Sarah Orne Jewett, Jenny June Croly, Mrs. Mary Mapes Dodge and others who have unostentatiously labored for the propagation of the suffrage idea . . ."

In 1896, Eliza was featured in an article entitled, "Talks by Successful Women" in *Godey's Magazine of New York*. Alice Severance wrote, "Among the noblest of feminine wage-earners are the journalists, and preeminent among them may be quoted Eliza Archard Conner, a woman of remarkable individuality, intellectuality, quick perception, and varied experience." She quotes Eliza: " 'Wait, watch, and work,' is my motto; the pathway of the woman journalist is beset with pitfalls from which only common-sense and determination and pluck will preserve her."

When Eliza's husband died in 1897, his obituary explained their living situation—he in Ohio, she in New York City: "Mrs. Conner . . . has been employed on many of the leading journals of the country . . . and has been compelled to make her home in New York and travel a great deal of the time." This sad and tender comment closed his obituary: "The Doctor was making his plans to move to New York, where they could be together, but death came and blotted out their plans."

James and Jane Archard's only son, Robert, was born on February 9, 1840. He died in infancy.

Daughter Laura arrived on September 23, 1841. She was a schoolteacher at eighteen, according to the 1860 census of Monroe Township, Clermont County, and married William Perry Flanegan in 1865. The Flanegans raised nine children: seven daughters and two sons. At least one child would relocate to Washington Territory.

A beautiful summary of Laura's life was written by Eliza in 1893 and published in her syndicated column, "Woman's World in Paragraphs," her instrument for informing and inspiring women across the nation.

"On a sunny green hill," Eliza began, "overlooking the Ohio river in Clermont county, O., is the home of Mrs. Laura A. Flanegan." She doesn't identify Laura as her sister. "Her husband's business keeps him away from home the most [*sic*] of the time, so the management of the beautiful farm devolves on Mrs. Flanegan." She elaborates:

> *There is scarcely a weed upon her farm. A herd of 70 Southdown sheep pasture in the deep grass . . . Dainty Jersey cows come at call and supply cream of exquisite aroma and golden butter . . . Flocks of chickens and young turkeys run . . . The rarest of fruits . . . shine in the trees . . . If you want fresh eggs . . . go out in the dewy morning and get them from the nests of the blooded [of good pedigree] hens.*
>
> *The home is a haven of rest . . . A rich, sweet toned piano is in the parlor; a library of the best books occupies one side of another room. Farmers and farmers' wives glance around this beautiful place and sigh and say, "I wish I could have things like this!" Then Mrs. F. looks at them and says in her quick, decided tones, "Well, why don't you have them then?" Sure enough, why don't they? If they had her industry, energy and brains, they could and would.*

The third daughter, Mary, was born on November 5, 1844, also in New Richmond. In the 1860 census, sixteen-year-old Mary is found as Maryn. Many errors in spelling are recorded on early census records, when the census takers wrote by hand the answers as they heard them. Mary's occupation is identified, along with her father, as a farmer. For all her achievements, she retained a love of the land and agriculture. Mary would wed

Edward Hempstead Latham in 1865, raise three sons, and earn a medical diploma in 1886. She would live an admirable, complicated, and noteworthy life.

◆——◆

Thirteen years would pass before James and Jane would welcome the fourth girl, Letitia, born September 25, 1857. Letitia is identified as Letty on the 1860 census record, at home with her parents. The 1870 census of Ohio Township, Clermont County, with a post office at Amelia, documents Letitia living with Eliza and her husband, Dr. George Conner.

Amelia, where Mary and Edward also lived, was described as an "old town" having "buildings erected . . . for a mile in distance, [giving] a straggling appearance, [and] residences whose style of architecture and attractive appearance is not excelled in the County."

Letitia married Thomas R. Cones the following year in Ohio. On their marriage license, she used the name Luie. They had one child, a daughter named Pearl. At the age of twenty-two, Pearl married Philip Richmond, owner of the O. K. Livery in Spokane. She would die in childbirth before her twenty-fourth birthday; but the child survived. Mary was the attending physician to record both the birth of the infant and, five days later, the death of Pearl.

Pearl's mother, Letitia, would use the name Louise once she came to Spokane to live with her son-in-law and care for her motherless granddaughter, Caroline.

By the time Caroline was twenty, she'd been sentenced to the penitentiary for grand larceny. Her name and mug shot are found in the Washington State Penitentiary records of 1920.

Neither her Great Aunt Mary, having died, nor her grandmother, Letitia (aka Letty, Louise, Louisa, Louie, Luie), were present when Caroline, sometimes called Carol, was sentenced. What happened to her grandmother remains a mystery. In 1912, Letitia's name appeared in Eliza's last will and testament, written as Louie A. Buckley, her address given as P.O. Box 265, Hillyard, State of Washington. Letitia's name is listed as well in Mary's obituary in January 1917, as Mrs. Louise A. Buckley, living at the New Madison Hotel in Spokane. Listed in the 1918, 1919, and 1920 Spokane city directories is "Louie A. Buckley, E. Longfellow cor [corner] Havana." In the 1918 and 1919 directories, Carol (undoubtedly granddaughter Caroline) is listed at the same address. In 1920, Caroline (in prison) and Louie both disappear from the city directory. It's been suggested that Letitia died as a result of foul play. However, her certificate of death was recently discovered; she died on April 3, 1933, at the Oregon State (Psychiatric) Hospital in Salem.

—◦—

The Archards' youngest child, Jane, called Jennie, was born October 15, 1850. In the 1870 US Federal Census, Jane is eighteen and still at home.

In the 1880 census, she is listed as Jennie Gee, having married William Raymond Gee in 1875. By the spring of 1889, Jennie had left Ohio with her family: destination, Spokane Falls. They settled in Washington Territory, becoming successful wheat farmers. In the April 24, 1889, issue of the *Clermont Sun*, a brief article reported: "A letter received from Raymond Gee . . . dated at Spokane Falls, April 8th, saying that they had arrived there on the 1st and were well and delighted . . ."

Most of the 1890 US Federal Census records were damaged or destroyed by fire in January 1921, eliminating the option of viewing family records for that year. However, an "1890 Veterans Schedule of the US Federal Census" for Spokane County exists, and lists "Gee, William R.," as having served in "the war of the rebellion" from October 2, 1861, until October 2, 1864.

The Gees' children were born in Ohio: two sons and two daughters. Sadly, the first daughter, Nellie, died at age six from croup, according to the US Federal Census Mortality Schedule. By the 1900 census, the family lived near the town of Sprague in Lincoln County, which had been carved from a portion of Spokane County in 1883.

—◦—

The Archard girls were familiar with the world of farming, and Jennie was no exception.

From Washington, Mary wrote to the *Clermont Sun*. "Speaking of wheat culture," she began, "reminds me of . . . a wheat farm of 1,000 acres where on one side of the field a reaper and header were at work—a steam thresher did its work in turn, while ten plows with three horses each were turning over the newly cleared ground for next year's crop . . ."

It's likely Mary visited the wheat farm of Jennie and her husband, about thirty-five miles from Spokane. A small news article in 1894 noted that Mary had returned from a "professional trip to Sprague." Apparently Mary had a close relationship with Jennie and her husband, Raymond. The previous summer, they conveyed a quarter section of land (160 acres) not far from Medical Lake to Mary, for the consideration (price) of "love and affection."

By 1904 Jennie Gee is listed in the Lincoln County roster of school-teachers as "Mrs. J. A. Gee, of Sprague."

The surviving daughter of Jennie and Raymond, Jean (spelled *Gean* on her death certificate) Raymond Gee, attended the Cheney Normal School to become a teacher. She wed Dr. W. F. Lamson in July 1909. He was "well-known throughout the state," and twenty-two years her senior. The newspaper wedding announcement described Jean as "one of the most gifted and popular young ladies of Lincoln county." Her father was not present at the wedding, having died in April. Jean would live less than four months following the marriage. Her cause of death is listed as "acute nephrits [*sic*]."

—◦—

Sarah Preston Baker Parker—daughter-in-law of the Clermont Academy founders—wrote an unpublished memoir manuscript about the Clermont Academy, in which she says, "[There was] an Englishman [likely John Archerd], a nurseryman who scattered all through the region excellent fruit trees. All the members of his family except the eldest children, James and his sister, were in the Academy. (When the academy opened in 1839, James was the eldest living son of John Archerd and his second wife, Mary McMichael.) All of James' family were in the Academy except one."

The education received at the Clermont Academy contributed greatly to the development of the intelligent, fearless, and compassionate women the Archard sisters became. Eventually the academy was renamed after its founders, Daniel and Priscilla Parker. "The school's founders not only believed in equality, they practiced equality in an era when that never happened," said Greg Roberts, administrator of the Village of New Richmond. The Parker Academy website adds: "In the midst of one of the country's darkest moments, the Parker Academy was a beacon of hope, freedom, and resistance, in a small town on the Ohio River that divided the North and South."

The academy also earned a reputation for being "the most thorough institution in the West for mental discipline."

Dr. Brian Hackett, of Northern Kentucky University (NKU)'s Public History MA Program, stated: "This is really what America is. This is the whole 'American Dream' summed up in one place, so early in American history. It was one of the first schools, if not the first school, in the whole country that was open to all races, all colors, all religions . . . It's likely that some of the people who attended Parker Academy were still technically somebody's property."

Sharyn Jones, PhD, joint director with Dr. William J. Landon of the National Science Foundation's Research Experience for Undergraduates, revealed, "We have archival documents that reference some students of color were the biracial result of a white, male plantation owner and an enslaved woman. Some of these men chose to provide a life outside of slavery for their non-white children and sent them from slave states as far away as Texas to the Parker Academy in hopes of preparing them for a better life than allowed for their enslaved mothers . . ."

An ongoing archaeological study hopes to discover proof that the Underground Railroad operated at the academy. Greg Roberts gave this informed opinion:

When interviewed on the subject in 1892, James Parker, the principal of Clermont Academy, denied participation while expressing his longtime support of abolition. There are other accounts from former students of the Parkers turning away slave catchers from their door.

Parker referred [a] researcher . . . to his brother-in-law, Thomas Donaldson, who lived on the adjoining farm to the Academy property. The Donaldson farm is a documented station on the Underground Railroad. Parker may have had reason to deny participation. I believe the Parkers directed freedom seekers to the Donaldson farm where they would be safe—just as James directed [the researcher] to Donaldson, where he knew any family secrets would be safe. Only dead abolitionists and Underground Railroad operatives were celebrated after the Civil War here in the Ohio River valley. Those still living faced possible backlash for agitating the peace and "causing" the dreadful war.

While Eliza studied at Clermont Academy, an incident occurred that could be considered foretelling of the ever-expressive girl. Mrs. Parker in her memoir wrote about Eliza: "The teacher made a radical change in the school; requiring entire quietness during study hours. To these changes she was not willing to comply. . . . She sat at her desk with her books before her from recess until noon, when she decided to leave school and go home."

Eliza did not return to the academy. However, "Some time [*sic*] after," Parker added, "when she had been a teacher for quite a while, she came to us to pay the tuition for a younger sister." Which sister it was who received Eliza's gift of tuition isn't clear, but it could have been any of the three youngest, Mary, Letitia, or Jane—although Mary had married in 1865 and was tending her home, while Eliza was teaching in Indiana.

Regardless of which sister Eliza helped to get an education, all five women led successful lives; their ambitious mind-set and dauntless approach to hard work seems to have been hereditary.

Following the death of Mary's mother, Jane, in April of 1902, an article appeared in *Our Mountain Home* of Talladega, Alabama. Essentially an obituary, the author, Mary Edith Day, wrote a remarkable vignette of the life of Jane Warren Archard, of the women who came before her, and of those she left behind. Day begins by telling how Jane's great-grandfather,

John Light, floated to Ohio on a flatboat, "Indians peppering them with bullets at intervals all the way and wounding Mr. Light himself."

John Light left behind his daughter, Mrs. Barbara Robb, a part of the Pennsylvania Dutch community. But not forever. "Barbara stowed away in a canoe," Day added, "her goods and her four children and herself, and in that frail craft they actually floated down the Ohio 600 miles and landed where the town of New Richmond now stands, joined Barbara's father and brothers, and grew up with the country."

When Barbara Robb died, she left behind her daughter, Letitia Robb Warren, who "was nearly or quite six feet high, strong as a man and gentle as a child. She was never known to be angry or to lose her head or her nerve. She was a famous farm woman. She planted fruits and flowers . . . reared a noble herd of cattle . . . [and] had great colonies of bees." Said Day, "This strong, gentle, fearless Letitia was the model on which her daughters and granddaughters built their own characters . . . Jane Archard's husband was much away from home on business, leaving her alone on the farm with her five little daughters." During the last three years of her life, following the death of James, Jane was the capable owner of the large farm. Jane was someone whose "Quaker ancestry . . . was not favorable to emotional fuss over things."

In closing, Day reported, "Of Jane's five daughters one is a physician, another a teacher, a third a newspaper writer, yet another a highly successful farmer, while the remaining one, now in private life, was until recently a stenographer and law reporter."

Without a doubt, Mary carried within her the genes of extraordinary women—"strong, intelligent, courageous and always cool headed"—and she would need every gene.

CHAPTER 2

Mary Weds Edward

SPOKANE, Washington, January 14 [1901]—To the Editor of the Chronicle:

In the first place, as soon as a young lady makes her bow to the world as a society girl she aspires to be socially prominent. Not everyone, to be sure, but we can safely say 50 per cent of all are recklessly ambitious to fortify themselves with a wealthy husband so that this may be carried on to the desired success. There is no thought on the part of herself or her parents as to whether she cares for the man she promises to love and takes for better or for worse "till death do us part." The solemnity of the oath cuts no figure. She is making a good match and the marriage is simply a means to an end. As the months or years go by what wonder that each wearies of the other and seeks solace and companionship elsewhere!

Another fruitful source of these troubles is the unhappy lot of our working girls, especially here in the west. Girls will come from respectable homes in the east where they were "just as good as anybody" and seek employment, expecting kind treatment from their employers, who in many cases promise almost anything and give almost nothing—certainly almost nothing of friendship and kindness, which these poor girls need more than anything. . . .

What wonder if this poor girl in her desperation accepts an easier life where kindness is offered? . . . [R]eformation must begin in the family circle, the home, in the public schools, and until it does, while we hope for much from the well meaning [sic] efforts, we expect but little until parents and those having young people in their charge come

*to the full realization of the fact that the children of today will be the
good citizens or criminals of tomorrow.*
—*MARY A. LATHAM, MD*

Mary wed Edward Hempstead Latham on July 28, 1865, at the age of
twenty, according to the Clermont County marriage license. They were
married in the Methodist Episcopal Church, New Richmond Station, by
Thomas C. Goudy, where Mary's great-grandmother, Barbara Robb, and
her grandparents, James and Letitia Warren, were members.

Julian Hawthorne, in his book, *History of Washington—The Evergreen
State from Early Dawn to Daylight*, stated that Mary and Edward were
married in 1870. These weighty historical volumes were not without error.
In fact, in Mary's own copy of Hawthorne's book, she took a pen and
crossed through the digits 7 and 0 in 1870, writing "65" above.

Edward was twenty-two, part of a well-established first family of
Ohio. In the "Catalogue of the Officers and Students" of Phillips Exeter
Academy in Exeter, New Hampshire, for the term 1862–1863, Edward
is listed as a Middle Class student, a designation assigned to students
enrolled between the Junior and Senior Classes, with an Advanced Class
being the final level.

By 1870, they had established a home near Mary's family. The Federal Census of Ohio Township lists Edward's occupation as a farmer and
Mary's as keeping house. Eliza and her husband, George Conner, are
listed as their neighbors.

Both Edward and Mary were active in the community—Edward as
a member of a fraternal organization called Buckeye Lodge, No. 150, F.
and A. M., and Mary as a charter member of the first grange organized in
town. Mary was elected its secretary, and a year later, grange master. Her
level of community involvement in Ohio was only the beginning of an
elevated life of service.

In 1880, Edward is listed as a US Storekeeper in the census for Clermont County. A news item out of Chicago in 1875 had announced it:
"Edward H. Latham has been appointed Internal Revenue Storekeeper
for the Southern District of Ohio." From early records it appears this
was a position of some responsibility. A US Storekeeper functioned as an

overseer of sorts for distilleries, as described in a historical study by the Internal Revenue Service:

JULY 1, 1880: Responsibility for the appointment of storekeepers, gaugers, and tobacco inspectors was shifted from the Commissioner of Internal Revenue to the Secretary of the Treasury.

JANUARY 1881: Beginning this month, distilleries producing 100 bushels or less each day were placed under the control of a single storekeeper-gauger.

Mary was still keeping house at the time of the 1880 census, but that wasn't all. Between 1866 and 1872, she gave birth to three sons: Frank (sometimes Franklin or Franklyn) Allen and James A., both probably named after Edward's brothers, James, Allen, and Frank; and, in a likely nod to Mary's mother's family, Warren A.

At the age of twenty-three, son Frank was a bit of a hero, albeit in a sad affair. On June 29, 1890, the *Spokane Falls Review* printed a correction: "The name of the young man that pulled the body of young James Fogarty out of the water was Latham, and not Leighton, as mentioned . . . yesterday." The body of Fogarty had been discovered by "two men . . . Eugene Eyl and Frank Leighton . . . [who had been] fishing. . . . Mr Leighton [Latham] swam out to where the body lay floating and tied a rope about one of the legs. The remains were then landed on shore."

Frank graduated from college, married, raised one child, and became a successful druggist, establishing businesses in Spokane and Tacoma, Washington. Frank's final place of business was in Seattle, where he often stayed in his apothecary on First Avenue, sleeping in a loft inside the store and regularly playing his banjo in the storefront.

Frank died—refusing to be seen by a doctor—twelve days short of his seventy-fourth birthday, with his son, Hesper, by his side. The death certificate lists the cause of death as "Senility."

⌐～⌐

Second son James became a popular union man in the city of Spokane. In March of 1898, his name was announced along with twenty-two other men who had achieved the level of journeyman plumber. In September, he served as marshall of the plumbers' union section of the Labor Day parade. By October he was serving as financial secretary for the Spokane Plumbers Union.

Everyone was "Fishing for Trout," according to the June 12, 1901, edition of the *Semi-Weekly Spokesman-Review*. Announcing who was going where for the sport, the article closes: "James Latham and T. Ashenburry expect to leave in a few days for Post Falls [Idaho]."

Early in 1903, James switched to railroading with the Northern Pacific Railway. It would be a fateful decision. James—or Jim, as Mary called him—was engaged, though he would not marry. He would die young, an event that brought great sorrow to Mary, Edward, and his brothers.

Warren, the youngest, led an interesting life. He also began as a plumber in his adult life, yet, according to Reverend Jonathan Edwards in *An Illustrated History of Spokane County, State of Washington*, Warren also served the community, perhaps following the example of his parents. Edwards stated: "Four young men, moved by a desire to help their fellow men, opened on the corner of Main avenue and Brown street a 'Workingman's Home.' They were Warren Latham, L. L. Dye, W. W. Gould and Mr. Warnell. They provided lodging for ten cents a night and meals for the lowest possible sum."

Warren married, and his only child, a girl, was born in January of 1899 and died before the end of the year. Mary would not assist with this birth. On the birth return next to the date filed, Warren signed his name, crossing out the initials "M.D.," and writing "Father." (In 1907, a standardized birth certificate form was developed. Before that the document was called a "birth return." All subsequent references will be identified as birth or death certificates, regardless of date.) For Warren, perhaps the infant arrived too quickly to summon help from his physician mother. Under "Occupation," he identified himself as a "Missionary."

In Spokane, Warren managed the Christian Home for Men, sometimes called the Latham Home for Men, aiding the poor, not unlike his mother. In December of 1899, Warren wrote a letter to the editor of the

Spokane Chronicle, asking that he "kindly state to the public that after nearly three years constant effort in trying to help those who could not help themselves, we are now compelled to discontinue our work for a few months." Besides giving their energy and much of their money to the poor, he and his wife were trying to recover from the death of their child. They were leaving for Pullman to do plumbing work at the university. Warren would eventually invent and seek a patent for a "farm ice machine." In 1933, Warren ran for the office of city commissioner of Spokane. He would live out his final years there, where he died at the age of ninety.

⌒

In the 1880 census for Clermont County, Mary was listed as thirty-four years of age. It should read thirty-six, according to her birth date. This would not be the only time Mary claimed to be younger. Twenty years later during the census of 1900, her birth year is written as 1854, making her ten years younger than her actual age.

Perhaps Mary imagined that by removing years from her age, her aspirations might somehow be more attainable. It seems she need not have bothered. She was bound for astonishing achievements. Edward would garner his own, first by attending the Cincinnati College of Pharmacy as well as Miami Medical College, earning his medical degree in 1884.

With their boys nearing adulthood and Edward having earned his credentials as a physician, Mary set out to pursue her dream of having a profession—in the field of medicine. Apparently, she was not intimidated by its vast scope: "The practice of medicine includes the diagnosis, treatment, correction, advisement, or prescription for any human disease, ailment, injury, infirmity, deformity, pain, or other condition, physical or mental, real or imaginary." In 1886, at the age of forty-two, she received her medical diploma from Cincinnati College of Medicine and Surgery, likely a student in the Woman's Medical College of Cincinnati situated there.

Medical societies were formed by the early 1800s, "establishing regulations, standards of practice, and certification of doctors." Society-affiliated training programs—labeled "proprietary" medical colleges—were also developed, eliminating years of general education and a "long lecture term."

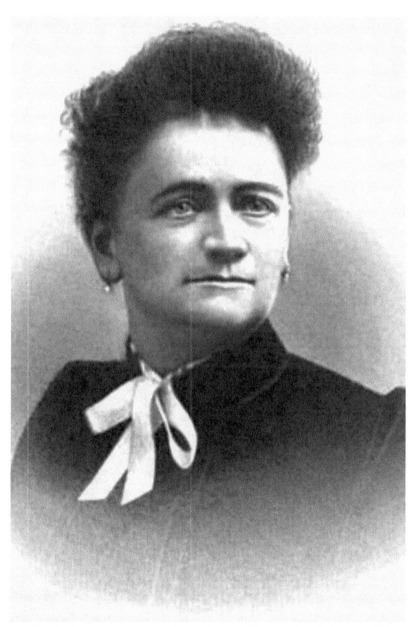

Dr. Mary Archard Latham, born November 5, 1844, in New Richmond, Ohio, died January 20, 1917, in Spokane.

PUBLIC DOMAIN

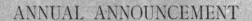

ANNUAL ANNOUNCEMENT

OF THE

CINCINNATI COLLEGE

OF

MEDICINE AND SURGERY.

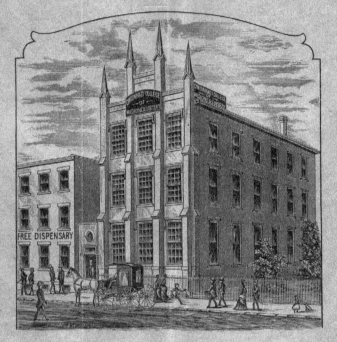

For 1880-81.—Forty-Sixth Regular Session.

MEMBER OF THE AMERICAN MEDICAL COLLEGE ASSOCIATION.

The Preliminary Course begins	The Regular Course opens
Monday, September 6, 1880.	Monday, October 4, 1880.

A portion of the announcement from the 1880–1881 session of the Cincinnati College of Medicine and Surgery.

COURTESY OF THE HENRY R. WINKLER CENTER FOR THE HISTORY OF THE HEALTH PROFESSIONS, UNIVERSITY OF CINCINNATI LIBRARIES

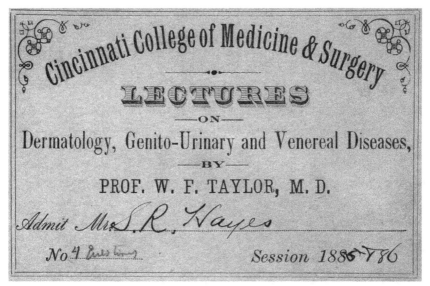

A lecture card from the 1885–1886 session, permitting student admittance.
Notice the word *Mr.* imprinted at the signature line.
COURTESY OF THE HENRY R. WINKLER CENTER FOR THE HISTORY OF THE HEALTH PROFESSIONS,
UNIVERSITY OF CINCINNATI LIBRARIES

One standard was added in 1852: "to complete a minimum of 3 years
of study, 2 years of which were under an acceptable practitioner." Perhaps
Mary's "acceptable practitioner" was her husband, Dr. Edward Latham.

Not only did Mary graduate from the program in 1886, but she was
also among the first class of women physicians allowed into the wards of
Cincinnati General Hospital.

Once Mary obtained her medical degree, she and Edward practiced
medicine together, uncommon for the time. Perhaps they joined forces
with brother-in-law Dr. George Conner, who was already established as a
well-known physician in Cincinnati.

The Doctors Latham were settled and prospering. And yet, change
was in the wind. Severe asthma, related to Ohio's heavy moist air that
made it difficult for Mary to breathe, overwhelmed her. She and Edward
began to discuss moving to the West, as proposed by her physician as a
panacea.

It's possible that in addition to seeking improved health, Mary may have been drawn to a place where there was room for her to spread her professional wings. The couple may have read the following description of a certain little village with a big waterfall:

The business interests comprise two banks, three wholesale and retail general merchandise stores, three drug stores, three grocery and provision stores, one commission store, two millinery stores, two watchmakers and jewelers, three gents' furnishing stores, four hardware stores, two furniture stores, three agricultural implement stores, three harness stores, three livery and express stables, three blacksmith shops, one machine shop, one carriage manufactory, two flouring mills, one saw, shingle and planing mill, one sash and door factory, four fruit and confectionery stores, two meat markets, one bakery, one soda water factory, one fruit nursery, one shoe store, two paint shops, four contractors and builders, one hide and fur depot, one gun and locksmith, three barber shops, two breweries, one wholesale liquor store, eight saloons, five hotels and three restaurants.

Spokane Falls appeared to have everything they needed to lead a contented and rewarding life, earning a description that could be used for Mary, as well—"an enviable reputation for pluck and progress."

CHAPTER 3

Climate Change

I came with no settled purpose except to get rid of business and hoped by spending a few weeks in dolce far niente, listening to the murmuring of the falls, getting where there was no sick person whom I had to look after, to find something which would make life once more endurable.

Eight months have passed and presto! the change! Asthma all gone, the strength of fifteen years has returned to me, and twenty-five pounds of good solid muscular tissue added to my former avoirdupois [heaviness].

Mary claims she will never live anywhere but in the West, and bears witness as to why:

There never were such blue skies and bright sunshine . . . and the water as it comes bubbling and foaming over the rapids, all the way from the snow capped [sic] mountains, is as clear as "aqua distillate," and just as pure, while the air as it comes down upon us from the pine covered mountains . . . is laden with a health giving aroma.
—MARY A. LATHAM, Spokane Falls Review, June 1889

Mary first sent this letter to the *Independent News* of New Richmond, Ohio, as a definitive and important testament as to why she had come to Washington Territory. She had begun: "Will you allow a former resident of your place to tell through your columns something about an as yet almost 'undiscovered country' wherein dwell many people from your county? [Others from Clermont County, Ohio, had apparently arrived in the area.]" Excusing herself for getting personal, she writes, "I came here . . . not quite a year ago, sick nigh unto death with asthma[,] . . . worried to death with overwork[,] . . . tired of everything and of almost everybody and having almost decided in the negative the question 'whether life be worth living.'"

Convinced Spokane Falls is the place anyone and everyone may prosper, "I believe," she writes, "that in no new city in the West has a poor man so good a chance in life as he has here. There are many good people here, and I think there is no state in the union not represented in Spokane Falls. Then there are the emigrants from almost every city on the globe. Iceland, Greenland, Norway, Sweden, Russia, Denmark, Italy, in fact every civilized country in the world has sent a number of its inhabitants."

She says she finds the men of the city to be real gentlemen, then addresses the subject of women. "There are many women here who like myself have stepped out of the beaten path in the way of women's work . . . [such as] May C. Jones, a lady minister, . . . Mrs. Alice Houghton and Mrs. Judge Bettis, who are large dealers in real estate, and very many others who are treated with respect by businessmen." She adds, "Gigantic business enterprises . . . [are] being carried on now . . . [and] numerous railway lines . . . [are] being built to and from the city."

Mary declares that "all desire for *dolce far niente*—sweet doing nothing—has left me long ago, and with ever increasing strength I am able to attend to business which is increasing in like ratio. . . . I feel sorry," Mary concludes, "to the bottom of my heart for everybody who cannot live in Washington territory."

It's unknown if Mary and Edward agreed to relocate to the Washington Territory, or if, taking the initiative, west she went. She was determined to live in the climate described as both *congenial* and *salubrious* in early accounts.

Several articles have stated that Mary came to Spokane Falls in 1887. It's possible these generated from the same source, Edwards's *Illustrated History*. However, no evidence has been found that she arrived in 1887. For instance, no one by the name Latham is on the census record of all inhabitants of "County of Spokane, Territory of Washington," conducted in April 1887. It did bear the name of J. W. (Jonathan Worthington) Scribner, who in 1891 would wed Mary F. Flanegan, Mary's niece. Also found in the 1887 census record were the names of the Doak family, including Howard, who would eventually serve as sheriff of Spokane County, with his brother, Schuyler, a deputy sheriff. Howard Doak would play a significant role in Mary's life.

Mary's name was also not found in the Directory of the City of Spokane Falls (1887). The 1888 directory for the city lists: "Latham Dr. Ma[r]y A, r 20 E 1st." The "r" indicates "residence," so it appears this was also her first home in Spokane Falls. While her first name was spelled incorrectly, the address is the same as the address published in her first medical advertisement.

Providing further proof that Mary must have arrived in 1888 is an article published in the *Spokane Chronicle* in 1894, in which a reporter states Mary proclaimed the prairie was soon to be covered by buttercups,

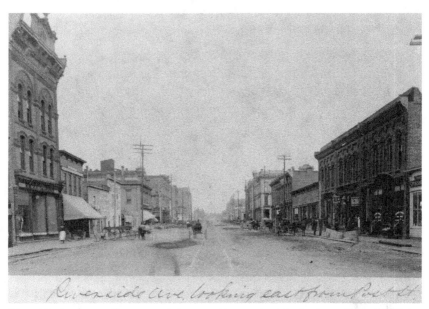

Riverside Avenue as it appeared the year Mary arrived in Spokane Falls, 1888.
PUBLIC DOMAIN

"a condition of things which Dr. Latham says has not occurred since her coming to this city six years ago [which calculates to 1888]."

One could speculate that Mary chose Spokane Falls specifically because a new-fashioned hospital named Sacred Heart had opened there. Though she came for a period of rest and to escape work, Mary must have known that the heart wants what the heart wants, and her heart wanted to practice medicine.

Sacred Heart was described as a "three-story brick hospital opened with fifty beds . . . [During] the first year, the hospital admitted 354 patients." This is according to Carl P. Schlicke, MD, in his *Medical Bulletin* article, "Spokane, A Community of Hospitals."

In 1890, a hospital for the mentally ill, Eastern State Hospital for the Insane, opened in eastern Washington. Deaconess Hospital's founding

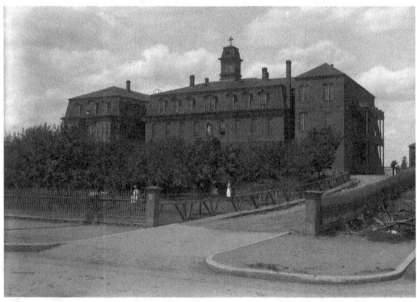

Only the central building existed in 1888, when Mary first attended patients at Sacred Heart.

NORTHWEST MUSEUM OF ARTS AND CULTURE / EASTERN WASHINGTON STATE HISTORICAL SOCIETY, CHARLES LIBBY COLLECTION, L87-1.1.3

was not far behind, an idea begun in 1896 when deaconesses of the Methodist Church rented rooms in a home at Third Avenue and Howard Street to provide a place for homeless and aged persons. By 1898, schools of nursing instruction had been established in Spokane. Schlicke states: "Deaconess [Hospital] was the first to initiate an intern training program in 1907." This was about the time Mary returned to Spokane after her unsolicited time away.

Also that year, a "Pest House" opened on the banks of the Spokane River to provide care for patients with contagious diseases. By 1910, St. Luke's Hospital, the Maria Beard Deaconess Home, and the Mountain View Sanitorium opened. Then, in 1915, two years before Mary died, the Edgecliff Sanitorium opened as "a special hospital" for those infected with tuberculosis. As a physician, Mary chose well coming to Spokane Falls.

—————

Mary's expected arrival in the West was advertised in a local newspaper in 1888, saying "Mrs. Dr. Latham will open in Spokane Falls, on or about the 15th of Sept. . . . a 'Home' where women . . . can be accommodated."

And indeed, on September 13, Mary placed a notice in the paper saying she would "treat free, until the establishment of the 'Home' for sick and friendless women and children, all poor who come to her office, No. 20 First street, between the hours of 8 and 9 a.m." Was Mary aware she had chosen a location within three city blocks of "houses of ill fame"? Perhaps she was, and this may be seen as the first evidence of Mary's willingness to care for the downtrodden of Spokane Falls.

Author Mick Gidley alluded to this announcement regarding Mary's arrival in his book, *With One Sky Above Us: Life on an Indian Reservation at the Turn of the Century.* He acknowledged that the announcement of her pending arrival helped to establish her identity and importance before ever lifting her skirts and stepping foot in the streets of the "large pioneer village . . . with muddy streets in winter and dust in summer."

In December 1888, the *Spokane Falls Review* announced: "Dr. E. H. Latham, whose wife has been here in the practice of medicine for the past few months is expected here . . . The doctor has been detained in Cincinnati, Ohio, winding up his business."

Eliza was impressed by the ventures of her sister and brother-in-law in the West:

> *There are great opportunities for women all through the Northwest. Dr. Mary A. Latham went a year and a half ago from Cincinnati to Spokane Falls, Washington, and opened an office. In the east she might have waited years before securing a lucrative practice, but in the young Western city she has already succeeded so well that she needs three horses to enable her to go her daily rounds among all her patients. Mrs. Latham's husband is also a physician, and the two are in practice together.*

It's reasonable to imagine the women of Spokane Falls awaiting someone of Mary's description: highly educated, experienced, and female—the first licensed female physician in Spokane Falls. Now, the women of the village could have their medical concerns addressed by a female practicing in the relatively new fields of obstetrics and gynecology, who would intelligently and empathetically—as only one woman could relate to another—attend to them, as well as their children.

Mary is further described by Jonathan Edwards: "Her learning and skill soon came to be recognized here and she has since steadily advanced, though she has long held rank among the foremost medical practitioners of the state. . . . Thoroughly devoted to her calling, and animated by a noble desire to alleviate suffering, she has always been a tireless worker." This book contains biographical sketches of significant citizens in early Spokane County, or, more accurately, the significant *male* citizens. Other than 10 women presented solely in a portrait accompanying the portrait of their prominent husbands, out of 890 biographical sketches, only 2 were of women. One was Mrs. J. A. Narup, a postmistress and owner of a general merchandise store, and the other was Mary.

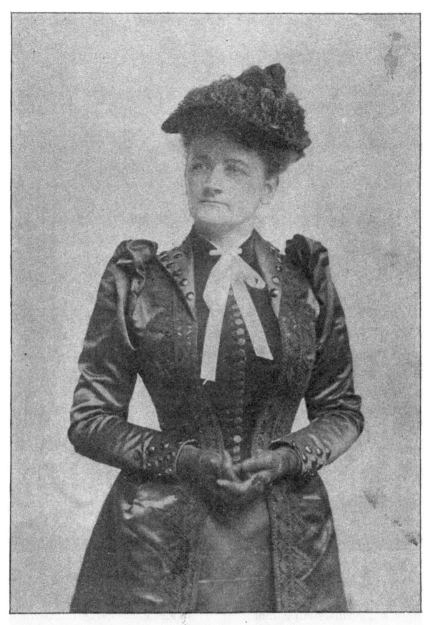

DR. MARY A. LATHAM.
(Photo by Maxwell.)

A professional portrait of Dr. Mary A. Latham in all her finery.

NORTHWEST MUSEUM OF ARTS AND CULTURE / EASTERN WASHINGTON STATE HISTORICAL SOCIETY, IMAGE VF-LATHAM.MARY.SR.1892001

In any far-ranging territory, "every homemaker had a do-it-yourself doctor book with instructions for self diagnosis [*sic*] and treatment," states Norman Bolker, MD, in his article "Doctors on Horseback: The Practice of Medicine in Washington Territory," in the Fall 1989 issue of the *Medical Bulletin*.

Fortunately for those early homemakers, in 1882, the Washington Territorial Legislature passed an act requiring those calling themselves physicians to provide proof: a medical diploma. Before that, anyone could hang out a shingle in front of their home or office and offer treatment. No wonder residents of Spokane Falls were thrilled to welcome someone possessing Mary's level of education. Besides having studied for and earned her medical diploma, Mary understood Greek and Latin and was fluent in the German language. And she was experienced, having practiced with Edward in Ohio.

Also, Bolker wrote, "The public was at the mercy of charlatans until 1907, when the Food and Drug Act regulating the safety and efficacy of medications became effective." The passage of this Act must have pleased the discerning Mary, although in 1907 she may have been too busy reestablishing her practice in Spokane to notice.

—◦—

Back in 1888, the village of Spokane Falls experienced a typhoid fever epidemic. Mary saw typhoid fever that year, as evidenced by her signature on a death certificate filed in December 1888. The fever finally abated when "the villagers stopped taking water directly from the river and began drawing it from wells tapping the aquifer."

Yet, much remained to be done to clean the waters of the Spokane River. For instance, a garbage ramp had been built at the end of Havermale Island, visible across the river from downtown. The island was reached by riding a ferry across from Division Street, or by rowing to and from the mainland against swift currents. Some thought it sensible and convenient to dump garbage into the river, where those strong currents, they believed, would carry it all away. Then, in the late 1880s, an important law was declared, which read in part:

No person shall place thereon or deposit in the water of the Spokane River within the limits of the city of Spokane Falls, or within 3 miles of said limits up said river, any hay, manure, vegetables, excrement, carcass, bones, meat, hides, offal, garbage, or any unwholesome or decayed substance whatever, or suffer, cause, or allow any hogs, horses, or cattle owned by him or under his control to lie, stand or remain in the water of said river within said limits.

Swimming, bathing, and washing clothes were also banned activities on the river.

Mary believed educating others regarding health issues was part of her duty. Nearly overwhelmed during the summer of 1888, she reported "a large number of cases of cholera infantum." These, she disclosed, were now mostly convalescing back to health from "a low type of malarial fever, which [I attribute] directly to the use of impure drinking water."

On another occasion, she warned her fellow citizens via the daily newspaper—perhaps the quickest way to reach the most people—that "an unusually severe type" of whooping cough was moving through neighborhoods.

In Bolker's *Medical Bulletin* article, he deftly described the medical profession of Mary's time, outlining how, in order to be prepared for whatever a pioneer doctor might encounter, her medical bag would have contained "scissors, scalpel, bistouries [a surgical knife with a long, narrow, straight or curved blade] for lancing boils, delivery forceps, hemostats, probes, ligatures and metal catheters." In essence, Mary needed to be a walking—or buggy-riding—emergency clinic.

CHAPTER 4

Big Ideas, Booming Burg

SPOKANE, Washington, June 9 [1902]—To the Editor of the Chronicle:

On Sunday, when returning from the country, and while waiting for a car, a bright girl 8 or 9 years of age, passing by, stopped and asked me if I were waiting for some one. I replied that I was . . . I asked her what she had in the pail she was carrying. "Oh, just some beer," was her reply. "Do you like beer?" I asked her. "Oh, no; I can't bear the stuff, put papa and mamma get beer every Sunday." She had been to a saloon, she said, pointing to it just north of where we were . . . and did I think it would do a mite of good and save this girl the trouble of carrying beer again, I would without hesitation give names, place and other data.

While on the subject . . . I wish to call the attention of parents and caretakers of children—girls especially—to the impropriety of sending them into the streets and blocks and all sorts of public places . . .

In the first place, if for no other reason, it takes away the modesty so beautiful in girlhood. In the second place, they come in contact with all sorts and conditions of men.

Referring again to the little girl with the beer pail on Sunday, at a time when the law says saloons shall be closed, I wish to say that I am not a prohibitionist, for the reason that I think prohibition an impossibility and am prescribing Spokane beer for a patient with nerve trouble . . . but would like to ask if there is not some way to enforce laws regarding the sale of liquor to minors, especially girls?

—DR. MARY A. LATHAM

Mary came to the West with big ideas and began efforts to implement them in her new hometown of Spokane Falls. Her actions were similar to those defined by Conevery Bolton Valenčius in her book, *The Health of the Country: How American Settlers Understood Themselves and Their Land*: "Movement pervaded nineteenth-century American life. Calling themselves settlers and emigrants, 'movers' and 'improvers,' households across the states and territories engaged in 'removes' and travels that reshaped the American social and political scene." Mary had removed her practice and home near the city of Cincinnati to the village of Spokane Falls, filled with determination to reshape her future, and the future of the place she would call home.

Almost immediately, there were accolades. When a local reporter decided to accompany and observe Mary on her daily rounds, this was the result: "Our pioneer lady physician is one whom Spokane may well honor. Her record as a lady and Christian, doing good deeds . . . is incomparable. The smiles that lit up the sad faces as I passed with her through the Sisters' Hospital [Sacred Heart] told more plainly than words can tell that she was a frequent and welcome visitor. Mrs. Latham is an earnest worker in home mission fields and never gives up on a good cause."

In the *Medical Bulletin* article, "A Very Brief History of the Spokane County Medical Society," Lawrence Pence, MD, made two statements that seem to perfectly describe Mary. The first: "Charity was an inherent part of medical practice." An early example of Mary's acts of charity was a dinner reception given in the city on December 31, 1890. "For Sweet Charity's Sake," read the headline, exclaiming: "Newsboys and Bootblacks Will Dine Free New Year's Night." Invitations were issued not to the affluent and prominent members of society, but to the newsboys and "bootblacks" of Spokane. "The dinner will mark the beginning of a new charity movement, instituted by a few local philanthropists, leading among whom are Mrs. Fowler, Dr. Mary A. Latham and Frank E. Doak." And the second: "Doctors were affluent and, in the public eye, revered." Mary's lifestyle revealed her affluence, by buying, selling, and developing land within and without the city limits. And by traveling extensively.

Pence ends with a question about doctors: "How could anything negative be entertained?"

Unfortunately, anything negative could. During the last dozen years of Mary's life, her fortunes would falter, and many dreadful and tragic events would occur—some entering her life through no fault of her own, others which she brought upon herself.

But for the moment, Mary was revered. Testament to that appeared in August 1891, when the *Spokane Chronicle* relayed this item: "This Morning between 11 and 12 o'clock, Mr. C. A. Gray of Medical Lake came into police headquarters, bearing carefully in his arms what appeared to be a bundle of clothing loosely tied. It was not long, however, before the officers and bystanders were relieved of any doubt as to what the burden was . . . an infant not twelve hours old." The bundle also contained a note with a five-dollar bill folded inside, instructing that the infant be taken to "Mrs. Dr. Latham," who would provide a place for it. She did, of course, taking care of the infant's immediate needs and later placing it in the charge of the sister superior of St. Joseph's orphanage.

—✦—

The following December, invited to speak in front of a gathering at the hall of the Good Templars, Mary delivered her essay titled, "Uncrowned Kings." Her comments included, "But God is not wearied with the type of king which each one of you before me to-day can make . . . He's a king—a true king, who dares do aught save wrong, fears nothing mortal, save to be unjust. . . . Duty is our ladder . . . [There is nothing] so kingly as kindness, nothing so royal as truth." Mary may have been a member of the organization, as the Good Templars allowed women members.

—✦—

In the summer of 1889, Mary joined a controversial new endeavor in Spokane Falls—the Northwestern College of Biochemistry, under the department heading Obstetrics. Known as Washington Biochemic Medical College, it was incorporated the previous year in North Yakima (now Yakima), a city situated about two hundred miles southwest of Spokane. Its mission was "to teach the principles of biochemistry and confer the degree of doctor of medicine on students who may become qualified." This new college was overseen by Dr. George W. Carey.

Biochemistry was a convention imported from Europe. In Washington, Dr. Carey gained notoriety mainly through his lectures. The *Spokane Chronicle* published one of his complete lectures in May 1891, which began: "Health is the normal condition of the human organism. To preserve this condition should be the high aim of the medical profession. . . . The biochemic system of medicine has opened up a new phase of medical science [that treats] disease with the inorganic cell-salts."

A lengthy lecture, it contained statements such as: "Dry mountain air, which is rich in oxygen, can cure ague [malaria or fever and shivering] spontaneously . . . Evidently dry mountain air is death on germs and should be named the royal germ killer . . . [T]he excess of water in the blood is obtained entirely from the air and . . . any amount of water we may drink can have no effect upon it." And this: "There is no specific diphtheria germ." Carey would eventually eat his words, for during this decade diphtheria was indeed discovered to be caused by a particular bacterial microorganism.

Nonetheless, he was adamant and boastful of his beliefs. "Let the sick bear in mind," Carey continued, "that there is only one way to be restored to health and that is the natural way, by supplying deficiencies through the blood."

He and his biochemic colleagues were quick to deride doctors in regular medical practice—meaning those who had earned a valid medical degree at a recognized school of medicine. It's interesting, then, that Mary associated with this college, since she was a vehement supporter of requiring valid medical licenses. This might be an example of Mary making decisions based on a too-quick, rose-colored-glasses assessment of people.

Carey's lecture ended with these words: "Close observation of little things is the secret of true science. . . . The truths of Biochemistry have taken deep root in the minds of thousands of earnest men and women in our grand, progressive state of Washington."

Or perhaps they had not, for *Dr.* Carey—along with a Dr. Reddy—was arrested and threatened with prosecution on a charge of "practicing medicine without a license." The biochemic medical college was short-lived in Spokane, as was Mary's association with the institution. Perhaps she discovered that Carey—ten days after his institution received its charter—had issued himself a fraudulent "registered" diploma. Later, she may have been referencing the college and Carey when she expressed her displeasure at those who perform as doctors without a legitimate license in her essay, "Women as Physicians."

In the *Review* in September of 1892, true to form, no reader was left wondering what Mary thought following the discovery of a pamphlet left in her office. In her essay, "Christian Science—Yes and No," this, in part, was her reaction:

"Christian science requires no faith." "Faith cure requires no science."

This word play [sic]—this "differential diagnosis" between the two "fads," "Christian science and faith cure," attracted my attention not long since, and the more one thinks of it the more there is in it, and the almost venomous manner in which those of the two beliefs try to annihilate shows that neither one has the true faith nor Christianity.

On the other hand, there are those among the Christian scientists whose daily life is lived in a way that the best and wisest of us might do well to take as an example, in the lines of whose faces as we meet them daily upon the street we read a lesson of physical, mental and moral purity, an expression of kindness and good will to every creature that lives, and unmistakable evidence of the genuineness of a desire to do some good to humanity.

"And you hope to bring about a new order of things by exorcising the evil and making the good take its place?" said I to an advanced Christian scientist not long since.

"My dear madam, that is not an iota of what we will accomplish. It will almost stagger you when I tell you what will come about, for in the first place all material sense will be destroyed and there will be no life as we live it now. There will be nothing left but the mind or spirit, the supreme, never dying ego, a part of the divine."

34

I wonder how we will all like that—this going about fleshless, boneless, garmentless—and I wonder how we will be able to recognize our old friends, for we will all be dressed alike in etherealism [sic], hobnobbing around in the empyrean [highest part of heaven], and the heaven of the Christian scientists will be here on earth also.

Some reports insist Mary was the first female physician to practice in the whole of Washington Territory. Clearly, Mary was, according to Pence in "A Very Brief History," "the first female to be licensed in the Washington Territory." One report gives 1890 as the year Mary received a license. The 1890 entry was likely a renewal of her license. Washington law required physicians to renew their license every two years on or before their birthday. Mary would have received her first license to practice medicine in Ohio in 1886; therefore, these dates falling every two years seem to further confirm Mary's arrival year as 1888. What is certain is that she is recognized as the first female physician to practice in Spokane.

CHAPTER 5

The Great Fire

This will not be a lecture on political economy, nor a lecture on any-thing nor anybody. I think that I have thought more seriously lately on the subject of money than ever before.

"For the love of money is the root of all evil," says St. Paul. As I quote this saying of St. Paul I find myself wondering how it is that I, an avowed disbeliever in creed or in anything that is tainted with creed, find so many good things in the Bible in which all creedists [sic] claim to get the authority with which they try to prove any dogma. . . .

Now about the love of money. It was the love of money that caused Christine [————]'s parents to send her into the slums and places of the vilest character, that she might pile up the gold for them. . . .

It was the love of money that induced the barkeeper where Tucker got his drinks to sell to the already half-drunk[ard] father more drinks, and in his drunken frenzy he made the atrocious attack upon his baby girl.

Again, it was the love of money which—indirectly, to be sure— caused the death of Lucy Greer, whose tragic death we are familiar with. . . .

I am not a prohibitionist, though long columns of statistics and long lines of figures stretch themselves out before our eyes in mute but eloquent appeal, and tell us that where one life has been saved by the use of intoxicating drink, twenty have been lost . . .

I am not a prohibitionist, because I consider prohibition, as the word is daily used—an [sic] Utopian dream [not until December 31, 1915, did Washington impose Prohibition], the creature of an enthusiast's imagination, an impossible problem, and all because of the moral cowardice of these men of the above mentioned caliber, and there are women, too, of the same kind who daily cry: "Lord, Lord," and do not the will of the Lord, but ask some other man to do it for them, for if they did it their customers . . . might stop their patronage . . .

While on the subject I will say that . . . there are within our gates other places compared with which a well conducted saloon is as harmless as a Sunday school. That is, if half that is told is true.
—MARY A. LATHAM, "The Love of Money—
A Very Good Sermon Written by a Woman"
(Sunday Review, August 16, 1891)

The above "sermon" was written by Mary two years after fire devastated most of downtown Spokane Falls and which, in its immediate aftermath, left most citizens on an equal footing, without the most basic necessities of food, water, shelter, and rest.

Midway through 1889, the year had been progressing as a promising, prosperous, and satisfying one. In fact, in January, the *Spokane Falls Review* had lauded the growth of the town through a letter the publication had received, "A Neat Compliment to Spokaneites [*sic*] and Their Enterprise." Written by Mr. Arthur Jones, newly arrived from California, the letter offered great praise: "Here is Spokane Falls, a city of 1,500 souls, built up in less than eight years. She is destined to become a populous city. Magnificent dwellings are being erected everywhere." Neither Mr. Jones nor anyone else could have known that *she* was first destined to burn.

That summer Washington Territory was experiencing unusually hot, dry weather conditions. A common topic of conversation might have been fear of fire. Regrettably, those worst fears were first realized in the "Great Seattle Fire" on the sixth of June, which hungrily consumed twenty-five city blocks, four wharves, and the city's railroad terminals.

On July 4, the "Great Ellensburg Fire" burst on the scene. This catastrophe was also called the "Independence Day Fire." Lurid flames destroyed over two hundred homes and buildings, including a ten-block area of the inner city.

As scorching temperatures and vicious winds prevailed across the state, Spokane Falls was not to be forgotten. Exactly one month after the fire that torched Ellensburg, on the evening of August 4, smoke was noticed in the city. While a lengthy *Spokane Chronicle* article would report the event, debate over who was responsible for the initial blaze continued for decades. The main assumptions of cause, however, were all centered on Railroad Avenue, where the conflagration was either started by a lunch-counter fire, by a kerosene lamp upended by a saloon girl, or by a spark from a passing train. According to the report, there was no panic at the first appearance of smoke and fire, as the threat appeared to be minimal. Townspeople believed the fire would easily be brought under control.

This perception could not have been more wrong, as explained by the *Spokane Falls Review* two days after the fire. While mentioning that spectators had assumed the fire department would quickly extinguish the flames, the reporter spelled out clearly how he had viewed the situation: "This [dousing of the fire] could have been done if proper precautions had been taken. But the superintendent of the water works was out of the city, and for some reason the men in charge failed to respond to the call for more pressure." It was later discovered the failure was mechanical in nature.

The *Review* assigned more space to extend eloquent sympathy to the other newspapers in town: "The sprightly and enterprising *Evening Chronicle*, the ably edited *Sunday Globe*, the old and well-known *Northwest Tribune*, the picturesque and hopeful *Graphic*, the serious and brilliant *Northern Light*, the elegant semi-monthly *Investor's Journal*, were all consumed in the flames."

In the space of an evening, much of downtown Spokane Falls vanished—more than thirty blocks that had contained edifices of commerce and places of residence. Flames hopped from one building to the next, fed by fierce winds and a profusion of stick-built wood-frame structures. The long list of sites that suffered complete destruction included the medical office and home of Drs. Edward and Mary Latham.

The *Spokane Chronicle* erected a large tent, assigning several employees to cover the aftermath of the catastrophe. These reporters assembled an impressive, many-columns-long, page-turning article describing the fire.

The article swelled with details covering specific businesses lost: Block by block, each and every business that had been reduced to embers was named; other details included the monetary value of loss, whether or not the proprietor had insurance, and if so, for what amount. Upon reading, it becomes clear that rarely had any business owner purchased enough insurance to cover the loss. Trusting in city leaders, and in the city's fire department, who could have imagined an inferno of this magnitude?

"The most devastating fire that ever occurred in the history of the wor[l]d, according to population," the lengthy article began, "swept over the business portion of this city Sunday night . . . At about a quarter past six fire was discovered in the lodging house over Wolfes' lunch counter."

The actual progression of the fire was outlined street by street, building by building, in an incredible elucidation of grand misfortune, beginning with the weather. "A strong wind was prevailing, . . . coming from the northeast and increased at times to almost a gale." It must have been a frightful experience to be caught in Spokane Falls that night.

Surely, city dwellers must have felt a sense of apocalypse. The fire spread so rapidly that then-mayor Fred Furth ordered buildings in the path of the fire demolished by "giant powder" in an attempt to quell the flames (a common practice at the time). This action further endangered the despairing citizens who were trying to escape the blaze. "The crowds at the reports [explosions] would start and run back," described a reporter, "and dodge the missiles that were hurled down on them from above." Additionally, "people were continually dodging the teams that were driving through the streets at break-neck speed." Sadly, some people were injured in spite of their best efforts to stay out of harm's way, and one person died.

The unforgettable spectacle must have seemed beyond belief, otherworldly, and hopeless. The dramatic telling in the *Chronicle* continued: "All along Post street were goods being burned that the owners had struggled to get out of their houses and places of business. It was now apparent to all that the city was doomed and all were seeking a place of safety."

In describing the path of the fire, the paper broke it down by sections—"Lincoln to Howard and Riverside to the River," for example. This part of the city included the Frankfurt Block, where Mary had opened her

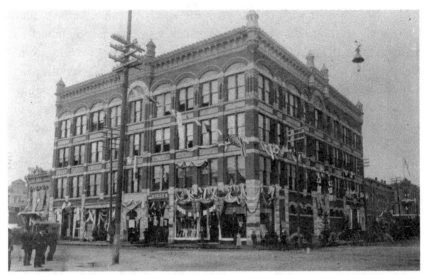

Before the fire of 1889, the Lathams' medical office was located inside the Frankfurt Block.
PUBLIC DOMAIN

office and welcomed her husband, Edward. "In a few minutes the entire block to the corner of Main street was swept by the flames, the magnificent Frankfurt block soon going down. This was a grand building, four stories high and covering nearly a quarter of a block, built of red brick, with beautifully carved stone finishings."

" 'A roaring whirlwind of fire' had reached the river and 'held high carnival' through the night." One can imagine a fountain of flames and sparks shooting into the night sky as the Howard Street Bridge over the Spokane River collapsed with a thundering noise.

In the aftermath, it became clear that every type of business required to keep a city functioning had been destroyed, along with many residences, all turned to ash and cinders amid heaps of stone and bricks. Guards were stationed throughout several blocks inside the "Burnt District" to keep watch over the various bank vaults that had survived the appetite of the flames, but now stood abandoned and vulnerable.

Mary was among many citizens already named in the article under the section heading, "Resuming Business": "Dr. Latham has removed

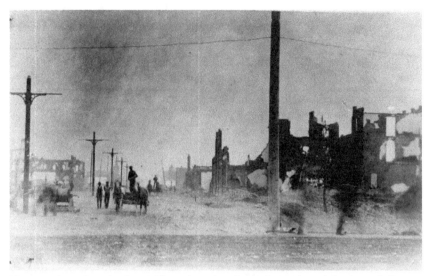

The morning after the Great Fire, when the skeletal remains of Spokane Falls greeted Mary and Edward.
PUBLIC DOMAIN

her office to rear of residence, corner of Stevens and Poplar streets [most reports cite Stevens and Sprague]."

In her "Woman's World in Paragraphs" column of April 20, 1890, in the *Philadelphia Inquirer*, Eliza praised Mary and Edward. "At the great fire in Spokane last summer they [Edward and Mary] were burned out of house and home, but immediately set up their office in a tent and proceeded to see patients as usual."

The fire that destroyed Spokane was newsworthy across the country. *Frank Leslie's Illustrated Newspaper* focused on what had been by publishing a drawing of Spokane Falls before the fire.

Newspapers in Los Angeles and San Francisco; Sioux Falls, South Dakota; St. Joseph, Missouri; Harrisburg, Pennsylvania; and Buffalo, New York—to name a few—carried headlines such as: "A Town in Ashes," "A

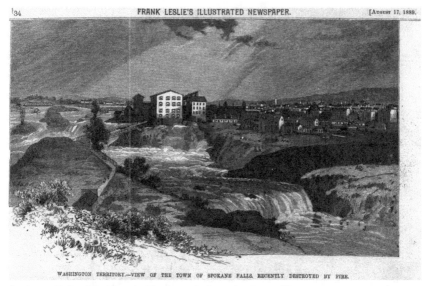

WASHINGTON TERRITORY.—VIEW OF THE TOWN OF SPOKANE FALLS, RECENTLY DESTROYED BY FIRE.

Spokane Falls, Washington Territory, before the Great Fire.
NORTHWEST MUSEUM OF ARTS AND CULTURE / EASTERN WASHINGTON STATE HISTORICAL SOCI-
ETY, IMAGE L87-1.41484-30

City on Fire," "Another Seattle," "Spokane in Ashes," and "Destructive Fire." The *Harrisburg Daily Independent* ran a small but telling item which included this statement: "Spokane Falls' great fire is a warning to all places where the water supply is short and the fire apparatus inadequate, no matter how large or small the locality." The population of Spokane Falls had learned this truth the hard way, even while living beside the rushing Spokane River. The paper's long report of the fire included a message to business owners and residents of Spokane Falls, set in bold type: "Let courage—courage, always courage—continue to be our watchword."

On the morning of August 5, the Spokane Falls City Council got to work, meeting with Mayor Furth. The following was immediately resolved: "That until further order of the council the chief of police is hereby instructed to prevent the erection of any wooden building without corrugated iron walls, or any wooden platform or any veneered building, except as a permit shall have been issued . . . [and that] the chief of police is hereby instructed to prevent the erection of structures of any kind upon

Lincoln street, Mill [now Wall] street and Stevens street, where the said streets cross the railroad right of way . . . [and] to use all the force at his disposal . . . to carry out the foregoing order."

The Council also adopted a salient motion that said "any person offered employment and refusing to work, be notified to leave the city." The mayor and his council showed foresight as they moved to protect the phoenix that would rise from the ashes.

"The city not only survived it . . . [the] holocaust spurred Spokane into a courageous, determined, far-sighted frenzy of rebuilding," wrote Rowland Bond in a commemorative piece that ran in 1964 on the pages of the *Spokane Daily Chronicle.*

Three months and seven days after the fire, on November 11, 1889, Washington Territory became the forty-second state to join the Union.

CHAPTER 6

The Doctor Is In

There are, at least, twenty-five hundred women in the United States who are licensed to practice medicine—there are more than that, who are practicing medicine without being licensed, and I have been cruel enough to wish that some of them might, in a moment of mental aberration, take some of their own medicines, and pass quietly to the finite quacks' heaven, or to some other place prepared for them. It was with a feeling of intense satisfaction that I learned on coming here that a physician must place his diploma on record, and be a "graduate" in all that the name implies. That was two years ago—in early times, when the city was in its "swaddling clothes," so to speak.

To-day, when the city has outgrown its long clothes, it is getting up a charter which is to make its framers famous and is putting on no end of airs, we see in letters so large that "he who runs may read" the signs of physicians and surgeons (God save the mark), who have no diploma, and who never spent a month inside a reputable medical college. (Allow me to say that this condition of affairs knows no sex.)

These quacks and pretenders bring ridicule and discredit upon those who are striving conscientiously to do their duty, and it makes a woman's progress slow and full of difficulties.

Christian, in Pilgrim's Progress, could not have been beset by more difficulties—real and imaginary—than we sometimes are....

I will say, too, that while the practice of medicine is uphill work, and full of responsibility, there is a delightful pleasure in being able to be useful and to feel that you are not living in vain.

—MRS. MARY A. LATHAM, "Women as Physicians," Spokane Chronicle (1891)

After establishing her practice in Spokane Falls, Mary offered support to her patients in a number of ways. Always ready to speak for a cause if she believed in it, more than once Mary would appear in court to testify on behalf of someone. One such case concerned Helga Estby, as told by Linda Lawrence Hunt in her book, *Bold Spirit: Helga Estby's Forgotten Walk Across Victorian America*. In 1896, Estby walked across the continent from Spokane to New York City, along with her daughter, Clara, during Estby's attempt to save the family farm from foreclosure. In 1888, Estby had been injured in the streets of Spokane Falls. For her suit against the city, it was Mary's testimony as to "the extent of Helga's injuries [that] likely aided the case."

Mary's next residence in the city—along with sons James and Warren—was listed this way: "rms [rooms] 508½ Howard," where Edward must have joined the family when he arrived.

The city directory of 1889 lists "Latham Mary A, physician 52 and 53 Frankfurt Blk," with no mention yet of Edward. By 1890, both doctors are listed in the city directory: "Latham Edward H, physician and surgeon Blalock blk . . . [and] Latham Mrs. Mary A, physician Blalock blk."

Interestingly, though Edward was listed in this directory, he was reported as having left for the Colville Indian Reservation, arriving for "the coldest winter on record there," stated Gidley, in *With One Sky Above Us*. When filing his physician's report to the Secretary of the Interior, Edward made the following statement: "It was in January, 1890, that I first came among them [reservation Indians]."

Yet, in March 1890, Spokane newspapers reported that the Drs. Latham had opened an "office and dispensary" on the corner of Stevens and Sprague, "at the rear of the former Louis Ziegler home." Perhaps Mary wasn't ready to advertise that her physician husband was no longer practicing with her. At the Stevens and Sprague location, following the fire, prominent citizen John Blalock built a six-story hotel and retail block, appropriately named the Blalock Building. This is where Mary (and Edward) were reported to have an office, even though they had separated. Perhaps the husband and wife attempted for a while to conduct a long-distance relationship. Occasionally, after 1890, Edward's name appears in Spokane papers, announcing that he was visiting the city and in which hotel he was staying.

In 1892, the husband-and-wife medical team advertised a two-room clinic: "Physicians and Surgeons. Drs. E. H. & Mary Latham. Office: Rooms 1 and 2 Blalock Block." Again, this advertisement conflicts with reports regarding Edward, beginning with his appointment to the Colville Agency. Of course, he may have used the Blalock Block office to treat patients who remained under his care for a time. Though he stated he was among the tribes in January of 1890, it was not until December of 1890 that a special news dispatch out of Washington City (Washington, DC) announced his appointment: "Dr. E. H. Latham, of Spokane Falls, was today recommended to be physician at Hespelien [Nespelem], Colville reservation." It was reported that he aided the tribes through an influenza outbreak in April of 1891.

Likewise, Mary was occupied tending to those under her care. During her first summer as physician in Spokane, she published a booklet entitled, "For Ladies Only." Inside its covers she provided instructions for women in what she called the four *H*'s: keeping a house, establishing a home, practicing proper hygiene, and maintaining good health. Proceeds from the sale of the booklet were earmarked for "the prospect home for women and children." This home-for-women idea would remain Mary's driving force.

By 1890, Mary was earnestly planning a hospital for ladies only—a maternity hospital. A December issue of the *Spokane Review* carried a short interview with Mary regarding her plans, along with another Spokane physician, Dr. Carrie E. Lieberg, to build a hospital for women. After remarking that she had received letters from interested women, Mary published her response: "In regard to the hospital, it will be built on the corner of Main and Post streets. It will be three stories high with a basement and the plans are being furnished by Cutter & Poetz, architects. We hope to occupy it early in the spring, but in the meantime are caring for a number of patients from this state, Idaho and Montana, and will continue to provide for all who come."

It appears Mary and Lieberg met their goal. An entry in the 1892 *R. L. Polk Spokane City Directory*, under the "Hospitals and Homes" heading, reads: *Woman's General Hospital—Main av cor Browne. In charge of Drs. Mary A. Latham and Carrie E. Lieberg.* Browne Street at Main Avenue is six blocks east of her original predicted site.

Curiously, Dr. Carrie E. Lieberg and the hospital disappear from the directory the following year. Mary remains published under the surname and physicians' sections. What happened to the "Woman's General Hospital"? One answer to consider is that the two women may have been forced to relinquish it during the financial Panic of 1893, when lending institutions called in their loans.

The Polk directory of 1895 lists Mary as a physician. In the 1896 volume of *Polk's Medical Register and Directory of the United States and Canada*, under the heading "Washington State Medical Institutions," is this: "Spokane Private Hospital—Established 1894, Capacity 20. Spokane. Physician-in-charge, Mary A. Latham. Matron, Miss E. Bauer."

In the 1896 Polk *city* directory, Mary is listed as living at E1122 Gordon Avenue—the same year that several birth certificates were signed by Mary, giving the Gordon Avenue address as place of birth. This E1122 Gordon Avenue address is not found in city records today, indicating that in the past there must have been a renumbering of residences.

—◆—

Mary's dream of a home for women having been realized, she called it Lidgerwood Sanitorium because it was located in the Lidgerwood Park Addition to the City of Spokane. It first appears in the 1898 directory with Mary listed as the proprietor, at E1024 Gordon Avenue. This Gordon Avenue address was on lot eight of land described as "lots Six, Seven and Eight in Block One Hundred and Eleven, Lidgerwood Park Addition." This was Mary's first Declaration of Homestead, No. 4205, filed on August 23, 1895 (she would file other applications in later years).

In 1899, 1900, and 1901, she remains at the E1024 Gordon Avenue address, but after 1899, she lists her office at 526 Hyde Block.

—◆—

In January 1900, an article announces the return of Dr. Carrie Lieberg, who "was in town several days this week as a witness in the Zienke case." There was a suit against Northern Pacific Railway, brought in November 1899, and was likely the case for which Lieberg was called to court, as she was "well known in railroad circles." She was "for six years, in the employ of the Northern Pacific . . . the first and only woman railway surgeon in the world." By 1904, Lieberg is listed in the city directory again, having moved back to Spokane to open a medical office. Perhaps she left for the railway job following her year with Mary.

Still practicing at the Hyde Block office in 1902 and 1903, Mary moved her residence to 318 4th Avenue, where her son James, listed as a railroad brakeman, also lived.

In 1904 and 1905, Mary opened a clinic and store and established her home in the town of Mead, Washington.

—◦—

By 1910, Mary had moved back to Spokane at 724 W. Spofford Avenue, still in Spokane, where she would remain until she died. According to the census that year—where Mary shaved eleven years off her age—Pearl Martzell, a twenty-five-year-old milliner, is living with her, identified as Mary's servant. This must have been an advantageous association, and Pearl more than a house servant, for Mary did love her hats. Similarly, Mary's sister Eliza boarded a dressmaker in her home in New York City.

—◦—

Despite her many moves, Mary was always ready when needed. Though she specialized in gynecological and obstetric care, she was available for any emergency. On September 6, 1890, one such emergency—thereafter known as Spokane's Deadliest Disaster—arose at the site of the new Northern Pacific Freight yards, where at least two dozen men in a construction gang were victims of a premature dynamite explosion. At the crossroads of Sprague and Division Streets, an embankment blew apart while the men worked. One might imagine Mary hurrying to the scene with her medical satchel, innocent of the fact that she was approaching the very spot where thirteen years later she would experience her greatest loss.

—◦—

Eight months after the horrid rail-yard explosion, Mary felt compelled to speak concerning an entirely different kind of death. It was the death of a girl, Lucy Geer (sometimes spelled Greer), whose name she mentions in her essay, "The Love of Money." Geer died following a desperate attempt to find someone who would end an unwanted pregnancy. The family's physician, it was said, had been asked to help but refused when he discovered the family had no money.

> *SPOKANE, Washington, June 25 [1891]—To the Editor of the Chronicle:*
> *There is only one extenuating circumstance connected with the crime of which Dr. Gundlach is accused, i.e., the criminal neglect of poor Lucy Geer, which resulted in her death—and that is the dread which any reputable physician has in getting mixed up in or being in any way connected with an unfortunate affair of this kind.*
> *There is always some one who is ready to blame the doctor for being the "party of the second part," who, after the girl got into trouble, took steps to help her out, and hence her death.*
> *But there comes times in every physician's life, when it becomes necessary to throw aside all precautions of the above kind, and risk reputation and all in order to do what the "unwritten law," which he subscribes to on obtaining a diploma to practice medicine requires him to do——save and protect life always.*
> *—M. A. LATHAM*

This letter to the editor is rife with irony. Mary has firsthand knowledge of the "dread which any reputable physician has" in relation to this kind of circumstance. And she knows what it means to "throw aside all precautions . . . and risk reputation . . . [to] save and protect life." As a physician, Mary will be accused more than once of taking that risk in order to "save and protect."

CHAPTER 7

Mary's Four *H*'s

SPOKANE, *Washington, January 29 [1898]—To the Editor of the Chronicle:*

I have wondered many times why those ladies, whose energy seems sufficient to "cleanse the Augean stables," [according to Greek mythology, stables that had not been cleaned in thirty years] do not turn their batteries upon the men, without whom, or [without] whose association, it would be impossible for these girls to be bad, and I believe that men would not be half so blind to reason, and incorrigible as women. And I am sure that I [could] say [to these women] without fear of contradiction that fully 90 per cent of all the girls who were ever once thoroughly bad, are irreclaimably so, and I will wager that these good ladies will find this more than true.

I had once under my care six young girls whose illegitimate children were born and had good homes provided for them. As the girls one by one left my home, I secured good homes for them also, and their past was as if it had never been. Of the six, five have now returned to their old way of life, the sixth having married the father of her child, who took her to his home, and in his manhood, has, as best he could, repaid the wrong he did to a good girl. The five deserted girls are fast becoming "toughs."

And what is the remedy?

Well, as we say in medicine, "Let it be largely proplylactic"[sic]— that is preventive. Let mothers begin by prenatal education of their offspring. Let it be a part of a teacher's duty to warn the young people, in no uncertain tones, of the danger of certain associations, and let the heads of families teach the same in home life. These and these only will lead to the hoped-for purity.

Going after these girls in this manner is like locking the stable after your horse is stolen, and while we hope for much from their efforts, we expect but little.
      —*MARY A. LATHAM, MD*

From her earliest years, possibly stemming from the moment she observed the terrible fragility of her dog Frisk's tiny puppies, Mary cared deeply for the plight of the helpless.

Keeping the helpless in mind, Mary was busy responding to her own set of *H*s —her favorite philanthropic bodies, which inspired, informed, and invigorated her: Home-Finding Society, Home of the Friendless, Horticultural Society, Hospital for the Insane, and Humane Society. Not surprisingly, she was a vocal supporter of each. The nature of her association with these organizations would change as the years passed, as would the kind doctor.

With an eagerness to help, make things right, and serve others, Mary became involved with a number of causes. Her home clinic received kudos from one Commissioner Parks in February 1897, when, after visiting Mary's hospital, he reported: "She is taking care of a number of patients and . . . everything is in first class shape." The "patients" were likely expectant mothers, wed or not.

Between 1894 and April of 1905 alone, Mary filed 166 Spokane County birth certificates for infants she delivered. Of those, only 4 infants were stillborn, and she delivered 4 sets of twins. All of the infants were identified by color as "White," excepting one birth certificate recording the birth of a "Mulatto" child.

Upon examination, these records reveal the wide scope of occupations of the fathers whose names were entered, such as miner, rancher, bridge builder, photographer, railroader, stenographer, clerk, bricklayer, merchant, musician, saloonkeeper, newspaper editor, soap maker, and tailor. These births as recorded occurred at locations ranging from her home clinic—listed alternately as Lidgerwood Sanitorium or Spokane Private Hospital—to the homes of expectant parents or other locales, such as Big Island (Havermale Island), the Hotel Gillette, and Cheney (a town almost seventeen miles away). Oddly, during the years 1893 and 1894, Mary neglected to fill in the name of the mother on nearly forty birth certificates. One might expect to see no father listed, usually in the case of an illegitimate child, but why no mother's name was recorded remains a mystery. One certificate had neither father nor mother documented.

A decade into living in Spokane, Mary's opinion concerning home-finding societies was published:

> *SPOKANE, Washington, March 11 [1899]—To the Editor of the Spokesman-Review:*
> *Referring to your article "All About Homes" . . . [I] will say that the ladies of the Benevolent Society are in the right. Persons adopting children (I have before me letters from six good people who would like to adopt one each) should be financially able to bear the trifl[i]ng expenses attached thereto, or be denied the privilege. Spokane has many benevolent people, in fact, their number is a legion, who have only to be informed of a worthy cause and their purses are open. The Spokane Home-Finding Society has in its short existence of a few months placed 13 children in good homes and has funds to spare.*
> *—MARY A. LATHAM, MD*

The Spokane Home-Finding Society (SHFS) remained a major focus of Mary's energy and attention. A short article in the *Spokane Chronicle* in March of 1899 echoed Mary's report, lauding the placement of thirteen children into good homes. Hoping to make it fourteen, the article ended with this: "They have one little girl of legitimate parentage, 4 years old, for adoption."

A year later, the *Chronicle* returned to the subject, raising the question, "Who Wants This Baby?" The many-layered deck (the subheads below the main headline), in bold ink, practically tells the complete story: "Detective McDonald Is Quite Sure He Does Not Need It—Dr. Latham Doesn't—Queer Way for a Mother to Do—She Was a Country Girl—Walked Into the Office—Left Her Baby Boy and Disappeared—It Wasn't Happy Till It Got a Bottle." The actual article begins with another question: "Who would like to have a little baby boy, 1 year old, dark eyes, brown hair, and above all a good disposition? . . . Any person wanting such a child could have had it free for the taking, on inquiring at Dr. Mary Latham's office on the fifth floor of the Hyde block today. Now it has been turned over to the Northwestern Home Finding Society."

The usual thing for societies to do was to place advertisements. The following September the *Chronicle* posted this: "Who Wants a Child? Dr. Mary Latham announces that the Spokane Home-Finding Society has two children for adoption—a five-year-old boy and a three-year-old girl—and that particulars may be learned at her office in the Hyde block."

In 1902, in an unusual article concerning the divorce of a couple, it announced the mother and three minor children were abandoned by the husband and father to fend for themselves. Having been granted custody of the children, the woman was unable to provide for her family. The Home-Finding Society had found homes for two of the children.

SHFS services reached beyond Spokane. Under the disturbing title, "Father's Alleged Cruelty" came a report from North Yakima, concerning a man who allegedly beat his children and was finally reported by his neighbors. The *Spokesman-Review* on April 23, 1903, said the man was arrested but then released, "providing he would turn the child over to the home-finding association of Spokane."

This article was missing something: There was no mention of Mary. Her son had died just three days before.

As the years progressed, Mary was still going strong, helping relinquished infants and children find homes through what she was now calling North Side Social Service and Home-Finding Society. This association was reported as meeting in Mary's home, where its members "decided to take up a campaign for relieving poor families and finding homes for orphan children."

A year before her death, one paper reported: "A baby boy for adoption, according to report of Dr. Mary Latham . . . at whose home the child is located."

The Home of the Friendless (HOF), a planned Protestant hospital cum orphanage, as detailed by Sue Armitage in *Shaping the Public Good: Women Making History in the Pacific Northwest*, opened its doors partly due to Mary's contributions. Eventually, Mary had something to say about associated events:

SPOKANE, Washington, October 28 [1902]—To the Editor of the Spokesman-Review:

While the controversy between J. W. Williams, the president of the Women's Benevolent society, the county commissioners, et al., waxes warm, I beg to contribute my mite. The taxpayers of the county may not be aware generally that their burdens are added to very materially by the help the commissioners are giving to the Home of the Friendless, the Home-Finding [S]ociety, the Catholic orphanage, and many and various others of their kind, which in many cases is all right, if carried out as intended, and yet not one of the above institutions is ever really willing to take a homeless child, unless able to pay for its keep.

Not long since I asked Mr. Williams to take a child whose mother was born, raised and married in this state, but whose husband got into trouble and had to leave.

He not only refused, but assured me that the other institutions would not take it. I referred the matter to the commissioners, and [t]hey assured me that they were paying Mr. Williams for "that sort of thing," and I went to him, with the above result, and I am now caring for the child at my own expense. My family being quite heavy taxpayers, I am glad this controversy has arisen and "got into print," so that I may be able to state the facts as they exist.

—MARY A. LATHAM, MD

Alas, the sadness continued in an article in the *Spokane Daily Chronicle* under the headline, "Terrible Cruelty." It was the story of a young Irish girl, Kittie, described as being among "a party of servant girls bound for Wallace, Idaho, where they had engaged to work in a hotel." Kittie "met a young Lothario, in the form of a fellow servant, whom she had loved more wisely than well." The article explained that her parents were well-to-do, respectable people, and that it was to "conceal from them her shame that she came to this western country."

Kittie landed in the house of a cruel midwife. Eventually, someone thought of Mary, who went to meet Kittie, subsequently taking her from the midwife's house and placing her in the Home of the Friendless.

In the fall of 1892, Mary came to the rescue once more. The *Spokesman-Review* ran a brief but descriptive item: "Dr. Mary Latham found a case of destitution in the Commercial hotel Monday." It was the all-too-familiar tale of a woman abandoned by her husband, left alone with her four small children. The mother was dangerously ill and the children were starving. Mary took the situation in hand, directing that the mother be taken to the hospital, where she was not expected to survive. The HOF took in the children.

To assist in keeping the HOF stable, in October of 1892, a benefit ball was held by the Ladies' Benevolent Society to raise needed funds. Did Mary attend? Was a *ball* considered to be without threat to public morals as compared to the "country dances" Mary would later condemn in a letter to the editor?

At police headquarters that same year, Mary reported a case of terrible destitution in an area dubbed "Poverty Flats." Following Mary's directions, police officers discovered two toddlers left alone in extreme squalor. The children were rescued and after the mother was located by police, she relinquished her rights, placing her children into the care of the St. Joseph's Orphanage.

St. Joseph's Orphanage, dedicated in 1891, was originally located "near the present-day Gonzaga University campus." Mary would often use the services of the orphanage. With the mission of the Catholic Sisters being "to respond to the needs of others, especially the economically poor, the marginal, and the oppressed," it's no surprise Mary would align herself with the organization. A Mr. Hoskins mentioned the orphanage when he came to Mary requesting she find a home for his two sons, who were currently housed there. Their mother had died in childbirth, he explained, and because something was going to happen to him, he wanted his children "in good hands" before. Mary must have assessed him using her practical physician's eye, for she later explained, "I told him that a stout man like him ought not to ask [for] charity for his children; that he should get his daughter, who is 16 years old, to come home, and then he should get his little boys and keep a home for all of them."

Two weeks later, when Hoskins returned to once again seek her help. Mary advised him that she had *not* attempted to place his sons elsewhere. The insistent man left, telling her she would soon know why he had asked this of her.

Soon the whole city knew why as well. Rather than accept the unrequited love of a young female Salvation Army worker, Hoskins instead killed her with a shot to her chest, after which he put a bullet through his own brain. Upon hearing the lurid news, Mary commented, "I believe that Hoskins had premeditated the act of Friday, and that he should not have been allowed his freedom after his acts of a few days ago." (Hoskins had been harassing the young woman.) Perhaps Mary regretted not acting on Hoskins's request; however, her assessment of him sounded reasonable at the time.

By 1894, the HOF was in the black financially, thanks to the contributions of the good citizens of Spokane, and the pro bono work of four physicians: Dr. Mrs. Hughes, Dr. Mary Latham, Dr. Fisk, and Dr. H. B. Luhn. This information is proof that at least one other female physician was practicing by this time in Spokane, in spite of Dr. Lieberg leaving.

An article materialized in the April 5, 1909, *Spokane Chronicle*, where the opening, long-winded sentence said it all:

> *The committee of citizens selected by the leading charity workers of the city to investigate and report on the orphan homes of Spokane made a report today to the trustees of the 150,000 club, in which a recommendation is that the "Orphans' Home of Spokane," conducted by Mrs. I. M. Day, be discontinued, and that the 27 inmates [term used to indicate a boarder] of that institution be turned over to the Home of the Friendless.*

The Spokane County Horticultural Society was another organization that benefited from Mary's philanthropy and leadership.

The Last Word—Mrs. Latham Asks All Fruit Growers to Make War on the Pests—To the Editor of the Review, December 6, 1892:
One more little word in regard to the woolly aphis and then let us say Requiescat in pace [Latin for "Rest in peace"]. Since my last article I have visited my orchard with a well-known fruit tree man, one who is not friendly to Mr. Genoways, and after going over 14 acres pretty thoroughly we found but a single tree infected.

I hope all fruit agents and fruit culturists will unite with the intention of ridding the country of everything inimical to the success of interests, for I believe that the raising of fruit is second in importance to only one thing, viz., the education of the masses.

Whether I am right in this or not I feel that it is the duty of all interested to see that "no guilty bug escape."
—M. A. L.

Fruit growers associations across the county were organizing into the new Spokane County Horticultural Society (SCHS). Names of men elected to office were published. However, the title of vice president was bestowed upon a woman: who else but Mary? She would also serve a term as secretary. Only one other member of the large organization was a woman, Rachel Grayson Creek. They were close in age and may have been friends, each dutifully paying their dues of one dollar per year. The two women met with the men to "discuss the different methods of protecting the fruit and trees from the pests that infest the orchards . . . and to further the interests of the horticulture industry."

Mary's horticultural endeavors were mentioned as a point of interest in a small article in February 1894, in the *Chronicle.* "Dr. Mary A. Latham and Mrs. A. Galland," it began, "have been added by Mayor Powell to the committee on reception for the Fruit Growers association. Dr. Latham has fifty acres in orchard now, and will plant an additional fifteen acres in small fruit as soon as possible this spring."

Never afraid to mingle with the men, Mary persuaded the society "to purchase quite an amount of flower seeds for free distribution to school children in Spokane." Mary believed that "as an educator and means of refinement leading to lines of higher thought there is nothing more useful than the cultivation of flowers."

That beloved flower, the rose, was celebrated at a local rose fair in the county, to which Mary lent her support, at least by donation, though she was likely a member. This was broadcast: "A handsome water color picture, the work of Mrs. Dr. Mary Latham . . . will be voted away this evening at the rose fair."

—✧—

The Hospital for the Insane (HFI) was another of Mary's *H*'s, located several miles from Spokane. This hospital offered a place of refuge for those in the Inland Northwest who were diagnosed as mentally ill. Eventually, the sanity of a certain citizen became a civic concern, leading Mary to speak out once more:

> *SPOKANE, July 23 [1895]—To the Editor of the Spokane Chronicle: Allow me to set myself right in regard to the affairs of Nancy Lammerhart, whose troubles it appears are far from ended. All I did in the matter was to vouch for the integrity of the ladies interested in her. There was no question of medical jurisprudence involved. No cunning lawyer was present, and if any one was paid anything we did not see the color of the money. . . .*
>
> *Mrs. Lammerhart is now in the city—as sane as she was seven years ago; is a spiritualist, which is, I believe, under our constitution allowable. All this ado about nothing reminds one of a remark made by a wag: "If everyone who is considered a 'little off' were in an insane asylum, there wouldn't be sane ones enough to support the others."*

A hospital for the mentally ill located in eastern Washington State had been an idea but nothing more in February 1891. Yet soon, the *Seattle Post-Intelligencer* had announced, "Proposals wanted . . . by the Board of Trustees of the Eastern Washington Hospital for the Insane at Medical

Lake" (located fourteen and a half miles southwest of Spokane). An article by reporter Jesse Tinsley in the July 4, 2016, issue of the *Spokesman-Review* notes:

> *Eastern State Hospital for the Insane opened in 1891. The grand structure was built on a "Kirkbride plan." Psychiatrist Thomas Kirkbride of Philadelphia advocated [for] asylums with long, meandering wings off a main building so that each section had exposure to sunlight and fresh air. He believed that attractive buildings and grounds were curative for patients.*

Later in 1895, Mrs. Lammerhart's name was in the news once again. Lammerhart (also spelled Lemmerhart or Lenhart) had been taken to the HFI following the death of her husband. It was then, her friends believed, that she had fallen under the spell of a con man—a Spokane-based spiritualist. The spiritualist gave a fantastic explanation concerning "a miniature railroad train, running on a track of wire." Longing to connect with her deceased husband, Mrs. Lammerhart went to see the spiritualist, who "assured the widow that her husband was aboard the train. This, he told her, was really in reduced form a great train that was circling through space, from world to world, with the speed of lightning. He demonstrated that its motive power was electricity and that a believer in spiritualism could travel without a ticket, provided the general manager received a tip in advance."

Somehow, Mrs. Lammerhart went from being conned to being incarcerated for sixteen months, until a court order freed her, following "the persistent importunities of Mrs. Ferris, Mrs. Mary A. Latham and Mrs. Sarah Vleit." These "importunities" were understood by the superintendent at the HFI, Dr. J. M. Semple, to mean "the representation of friends that she would be taken care of." However, he made it clear when he released the patient that he believed "she is crazy yet." Dr. Semple continued, "Of the women connected with the case, Dr. Mary Latham went no further than to certify that the other two [Ferris and Vleit] were proper persons."

A piece about Mary—"She Is a Deputy Sheriff"—appeared in the *Spokane Chronicle* in April of 1896.

This morning Dr. Mary A. Latham was deputized to act as a deputy sheriff by Officer Deputy Maguire, the doctor appointed an escort to Mrs. Arnold, wife of a well known [sic] printer, who was examined as to her sanity and sentenced to Medical Lake asylum. Deputy Maguire says this is the first time a woman was ever deputized in the state and is the second instance in the west, a lady having previously been appointed a deputy in Wyoming. Mrs. Arnold, who is the mother of a large family of children, has been an invalid for some years, and has shown decided signs of mental weakness during the past few days.

Only four years later, Mary was instrumental in having a different woman committed. A five-line article read: "Sent to the Asylum—The examination of Mrs. Susan T. Glover yesterday afternoon resulted in her being declared insane by Drs. Freeman and Mary Latham, and she was committed to the asylum at Medical Lake by Judge Richardson." Susan T. Glover was the wife of James Glover, an early pioneer dubbed "The Father of Spokane." Regardless of Mary's faith in her diagnosis after examining Mrs. Glover, she, as an intelligent, industrious, independent, and freedom-loving woman, must have been aggrieved to some measure to send another woman away from family and friends to be locked inside an institution.

—◆—

The Humane Society of Spokane (HSS)—her final *H*—was very important to Mary.

THE LEAST OF THESE – A Plea for the Humane Society of Spokane Falls, February 9, 1890 — To the Editor of the Review:
"Inasmuch as ye have done it to the least of these, my little ones, ye have done it unto me." In these words so full of pathetic mourning and pleading does the great power of humanity, whose kindly spirit is in sympathy with every effort for good, ask for the cooperation of all mankind for the weak and helpless of earth.

Who are the "least of these"?

Verily, their name is legion—they are many in our city, though benevolent societies are being organized on every hand....

A little boy of not more than 9 years was sent from his home at midnight, during the recent severely cold weather, to sell morning papers....

Little girls of 7 and 10 are sent to sell evening papers in places where scenes are enacted which would make a fiend incarnate blush for shame ...

A cripple girl is sent on pleasant afternoons to sell flowers, and, like the newsboy, uses her deformity to excite pity and draw trade ...

Dumb beasts are left standing in from four to six inches of water, tied fast beyond all hope of escape; cold, hungry, thirsty ...

Yet there are those who ridicule the idea of a Humane Society in our city ...

Where, in all the wide field of literature, sacred or secular, can you find any four words which mean so much as these: "Thy neighbor as thyself." Who is my neighbor? Every living creature that treads the earth is our neighbor.

Then may we not have the help of every intelligent person in Spokane Falls in our newly organized Humane Society?

The work here is great, and the laborers as yet are few.

—M. A. LATHAM

As humane societies were shaped across the nation, the aim of each organization was to assist not only helpless animals on the street, but also children and others in desperate need.

"American Humane [the country's first national humane organization] was founded," according to *American Humane*, "on October 9, [1877], in Cleveland, Ohio, by local humane society representatives from around the United States. The new organization's first goal was to secure humane treatment for working animals and livestock in transit."

In Spokane, after listing newly elected officers of the HSS, including treasurer Mary, the purpose of the organization was described in the *Spokane Chronicle* of May 13, 1891: "The work of the organization is in all lines by which humanity may be benefitted [*sic*], especially the prevention of cruelty to children and animals and the suppression of vice." One month later, Mary would become president of the society.

And yet, on May 17, 1896, a curious article titled "To Organize a Humane Society" appeared. It began, "A number interested in the organization of a humane society met last evening at the office of Mary A. Latham." In the 1896 issue of the *R. L. Polk & Co., Spokane City Directory*, "Mary A. Latham" is listed as president of the Spokane Branch Humane Society. Perhaps that first announced formation of a humane society in Spokane failed and citizens were eager to try again. Or perhaps they chose to separate themselves from a certain member of the first organization: the infamous Dr. Carey.

In addition to Mary, Mrs. H. J. Cook, H. N. Maguire, Mrs. Irons, and H. W. Andrews were also in attendance, discussing how "strong and influential societies exist[ed] in all the great cities" and how the state organizations served as an "auxiliary to the American Humane Society." Those gathered remarked that the membership consisted of "the most prominent and influential men and women of the nation."

Moving forward, this group of concerned citizens were elated that legislation had passed with the aim of preventing "Cruelty to domestic animals and wanton destruction of animal life of any kind by sportsmen and others." At this meeting, several speakers urged the formation of a society for the protection of animals. Mary stepped to the podium, hoping to persuade attendees "that some society that would be active in its work and fill the place should be organized at once."

The meeting was a success. On May 24, 1897, an incorporation meeting was held where eighteen Spokane residents attended as charter members, Mary among them. Three years later, R. J. Hanlon, "public relations expert, headquartered with the national humane organization in Milwaukee, had been stumping his way west." He stopped to speak to the Spokane branch, in part saying, "The object of the association is primarily to prevent cruelty of parent toward child and of owner toward beast. . . . People who cruelly treat their own children and those in their care should be given to understand that such conduct will not be tolerated in a civilized community." One might imagine the stalwart Mary nodding her head in emphatic agreement.

CHAPTER 8

Essayist Extraordinaire

SPOKANE, Washington [March 17, 1891]—To the Editor of the Review:

You christened my article in last Sunday's Review "Views of a Skeptic," after I had already named it "How Skeptics Are Made." Now, I am not a skeptic as the word goes—[I] am only skeptical in regard to the genuineness of the religion of a person who sins for six days out of seven, and on the seventh day, with elongated face and sanctimonious air, enters the church, occupies a front seat, on being called upon to lead in prayer will tell the Lord what the Lord's duty is, and ask him to make the whole world believe just as he believes, so that they may have a ghost of a chance to enter the golden gate, after he himself has entered and selected the best seat. This man's conscience has not allowed him to have a sound night's sleep for years, yet for fifty-two days in the year he goes through the solemn mockery.

Some one said to me yesterday, "Why do you dislike ministers so much?" I do not dislike ministers, and I know of many in this city to-day who are going about doing the Master's work with an earnestness of purpose and genuineness of heart that there can be no mistaking, but candor compels me to say that in my business, which takes me alike into the houses of rich and poor, I have met at the bedside of the sick and dying twice as many of the Roman Catholic clergy as of the Protestant clergy, and not only did they give spiritual consolation to the sin-burdened soul, but food and clothing, and attended to the temporal wants of the sufferer with as much kindly tenderness as a sister [nun].

"By their fruits ye shall know them," and I am skeptical of all who show no fruits. . . .

Let us stop quarreling over all these questions which are too great for the human mind in its present status to unravel, do all the good we can, do as little harm as possible for erring nature to do, and trust to the power who sent us to an existence here.

—MARY A. LATHAM

As a prolific author of essays, short stories, and frequent letters to the editors of several newspapers, Mary's skill with the pen gained in reputation from her first days in the community. In December 1890, the *Spokane Falls Review* received a request: "Please publish in your next issue the name of the author of the story in the Christmas *Review* called 'A Queer Mascot.' We have been guessing and want to know who he is." Here, it's obvious the reader assumed the story was written by a man. The editor responded using brackets: "[By an oversight the name of the author was omitted in publication. The pathetic little story was written by Mrs. Dr. Mary A. Latham, of this city.]" Surely, the editor is implying the sad plot of the story, not Mary's skill as a writer.

Following is the brief story as published on Christmas Day, 1890:

"Yes, the price has riz, and you can't git one, not for less'n six bits. Ye should a' took one this mawnin' when you could a' got one, for fo'."

The speaker was a grocery man, the person spoken to was "Speckie," whose line of beauty was almost obliterated by numerous freckles, and a shock of red brown hair which crowned his head, but there was no mistaking the honesty that shone out from his bright blue eyes.

Speckie's heart went down to zero, so to speak, when told that the price of the Christmas fowls with which he hoped to surprise his mother and invlid [sic] sister was beyond his reach.

He had worked selling papers, early and late, had denied himself his bun and coffee that morning, but his hungar, [sic] his cold feet, and mittenless [sic] hands, all seemed as nothing, as he looked forward to the good dinner they would have when he got home that night.

"Two bits more, two bits more. How shall I get them?" he kept asking. Speckie started out again, found a load of coal to put in—the man was in a hurry—could not stop to get change, gave him 15 cents and hurried away.

"Ten cents more, 10 cents more. How shall I get it?"

Speckie past [sic] the grocer's to see if the coveted fowl was still there—only two left—the best one was gone.

Again he started out; it was too late to risk any money on papers. He could see hotel waiters, fat and saucy, carrying trays of savory dinners to people who never had known what it was to feel hungry.

Rich ladies, dressed in furs and costly raiment, with glistening diamonds, passed him on their return from church, where they had heard anew the old, old story of the Christ-child, and listened to such an affecting sermon that they had given a few extra dollars to swell the minister's already liberal collection. "They felt so comforted by his words," they said. This minister was young, popular and unmarried.

"Only 10 cents more, only 10 cents more," and Speckie stopped a minute to look at the heaps of gold just inside the banker's window. Just next door he could hear the chink of the change as the saloonkeeper raked in the dollars.

"Ten cents more, 10 cents more," he kept saying. "How shall I get it?"

Speckie again peeped into the grocer's window—only one chicken left—the smallest one and in a half hour the grocer said he would close.

"Can I carry your valise for you?" he asked of a gentleman passing. "I will carry it as far as you wish for 10 cents," and taking the valise, so heavy a one, that he staggered with its weight, he started. "Only 10 cents more, and I'll soon get it," said the hopeful Speckie.

The weary tramp at last ended and he ran joyfully to the grocer's. It was snowing now, and the snow stuck to the poor boy's thinly-clad feet, hung on his red brown hair, trickled down his neck, but he ran on so earnestly that he did not hear the loud shouts of a tall man well dressed [sic] except that he wore a broad "cowboy" hat and high top [sic] boots. The man started to overtake Speckie, but so fleet was he, filled as he was with alternate hope and fear, in regard to his Christmas dinner, that the attempt was useless.

"Well, kid, yer back fer yer chicken, air yer?" said the grocer, who was just tying the chicken up to take to his own home.

"I reckoned I couldn't sell it and thought I'd rather eat it myself than to hev it spile, but ef you've got yer 6 bits ye kin hev it."

Speckie spread, with his stiff, cold fingers, the coins upon the counter, and started to the door feeling that now no earthly power could rob him of the prize of which he had worked so hard to win.

"Here, you confounded little jackanapes, you, this is what ye've bin a-snoopin' around all day fer, is it? I 'spicioned ye wasn't no good when I see ye peekin' in," shrieked the grocer.

"Is there not money enough? There are 6 bits," Speckie tried to say.

"Come off now, and don't ye try to make me think ye didn't know that fo' bits piece was the commonest kind o' pewter. Just ye lay that there fowl down an' take yer money and git an' be glad I don't run ye in, which I'd do in a minute if I had time to spare to report ye."

Poor Speckie picked up his coins, started for the door, slipped on the steps, reeled, fell—his arm was broken, the money rolled into the muddy snow on the sidewalk, and—"Well, I've caught up with you at last," said the tall man with the cowboy hat and high top boots, who came hurrying up. "Here, kid, I made a mistake, and gave you a bad half-dollar this morning. I want it. Here is a dollar for it."

But Speckie said never a word. Cold, hunger, fright and pain had been mercifully relieved, for the poor fellow had fainted.

"What's this all about, mister?" said he to the grocer.

"Well, it's just this. That there kid—he's been snoopin' 'round here purty near all day, a-askin' the price o' my fowls, and I sold him the last one I had, and he gimme a pewter fo'-bit piece, and I took the chicken, an' told him to git, an' I reckon he must a fell, and I reckon we better send fur a cop to take him somewhere."

Tenderly picking up the senseless boy, and securing the coin, which still lay in the muddy snow, Mr. Gregory, for such was his name, carried him away from the scene of the trouble. Where to take him he did not know.

But he did know that somewhere in the wide world he had a son, and maybe that some one [sic] would on this Christmas day be kind to *him. After a short time Speckie opened his eyes and asked: "Are you a policeman? Oh, no! I see now. You are the man who gave me the bad half dollar. I'm sure you did not know it was bad, did you?"*

"Tell me where you live, sonny, and I will take you home, as your arm is broken and I'm afraid you can not [sic]walk."

A carriage was called, a surgeon ordered, to the number in "G" alley which Speckie gave, and on the way he told Mr. Gregory as much as he knew of his very early life, when he had a father, a good home, how his father had gone, when his little sister was a baby, to the West, and intended to send for his family.

This he did but after coming to the West they could not find him, and grew poorer and poorer. How he had worked and gone hungry that day, in order to give his mother and sister a pleasant surprise.

"And, mister," he continued, "please try and not notice how poor we are, for it would distress Mother, and she works so hard and does the best she can with what we have in our house."

Up a rickety stairway, down a long, dark hallway Gregory carried his burden. Something, he could not tell what, caused him to go so lightly that his approach was not noticed. Glancing through a little window he saw a woman and little girl, pale with long sickness and poverty.

"Mamma," he heard the little one say, "I dreamed that Santa Claus came to our house, but he did not look at all like the Santa Claus we see in the pictures, and Mamma, I'm just as sure as I can be that we will have a pleasant Christmas yet, though it is already dark; and Mamma, I am so hungry, but it will not be for long."

A knock, to which the mother responded, was heard, and Mr. Gregory, carrying his helpless burden, followed by the surgeon, entered.

Laying the tired little body of Speckie upon a couch, Gregory turned to address the boy's mother.

A long earnest look, and "Oh! Margaret, can it be that I have found you, and in this place? Will God ever forgive me?"

"Oh! Robert, my husband, my darling, am I not dreaming? Only just now Nellie told me that she knew that Santa Claus would come."

The surgeon had dressed the broken arm in some mysterious way. A message had been sent out, and package after package of food, clothing and all good things came to the little home in "G" alley.

In the morning a carriage for the family and a wagon for the few movables came, and the little home knew them no longer. Instead we see them in a cosy [sic] home, surrounded by all the comforts and many luxuries.

Gregory had come to the West, had struck it rich, had sent for his family, but in the confusion that sometimes occurs in the new West, a mistake had been made, and they became lost.

The pewter half dollar had been useful to him more than once, and he had carried it as a "pocket piece" for years, and he has never been able to explain how he came to make the mistake which led him to find his family.

Upon examination, it's clear that the themes woven into the fabric of the tale reflect the author's life experiences. For example, the hero of the story traveled to the West, established himself well, sent for his family, but then they were lost. Mary came to the West, established herself well by becoming a revered physician, and waited for her husband to join her. Of course, Mary's story does not contain a happy marital ending akin to the joy experienced by little Speckie's parents.

Furthermore, at a crucial point in the story a surgeon was called who cared for the injured child "in some mysterious way." This seems to echo Mary's caring for the children of the city. She is also teaching moral values. Speckie, the protagonist, practices thoughtfulness and self-sacrifice in his quest for the surprise—a nurturing gift of food—for his mother and suffering sister. He perseveres past many hardships to attempt to accomplish his goal of purchasing a fowl for dinner. He is honest—so honest that it "shone out" from his blue eyes. The cowboy with the high boots practiced kindness by looking for the boy so he could make amends for his mistake, going beyond what might have been expected by offering the boy a dollar to replace a fifty-cent piece.

This may have been how Mary—honest, thoughtful, and kind to her patients—felt when she persevered, vanquishing a number of obstructions placed in front of women in her time, working long and hard over several years to accomplish her goals.

The cleverness and poignancy of this compact story demonstrates that Mary was a natural writer. It's possible that becoming a published writer was one of her goals. It was definitely one of the many skills at which she excelled. She learned early the power of the pen. Mary's sister, Eliza, by then of New York City, was a prolific writer and journalist, catering to women's issues. Eliza's well-known endeavor, "Woman's World in Paragraphs," appeared in an astounding number of newspapers and magazines. In the April 20, 1890, issue of the *Philadelphia Inquirer*, Eliza, in her essay entitled, "Work, Will and Wait—The Changed Ideal of Feminine Beauty," states, "The change in the ideal of feminine beauty in the last generation is striking." She describes how now, rather than dainty, swan-like images of the past, the ideal woman "has square shoulders, a full neck, a flat back, and carries her head erect." It's as if Eliza were describing Mary. L. E. Bragg, in her book, *More Than Petticoats: Remarkable Washington Women*, describes Mary similarly. "Standing 5' 6" tall, erect of carriage, with brown hair, blue eyes, and angular features, Mary exuded dignity, pride, and professionalism."

CHAPTER 9

Child Care

SPOKANE, Washington, August 10 [1891]—To the Editor of the Chronicle:

Is there, in this city, a kindergarten school? If so, will you kindly tell the public where it is and by whom kept? Many persons have lately inquired for one and so far I have failed to get any information that is satisfactory.

If there is not one, I would suggest that some lady who understands the kindergarten work, start one, it will surely pay so far as money goes, and it will give many a working woman a chance to put her little ones in good hands while at work through[ou]t the day.

Very truly,

—MARY A. LATHAM

Spokane County records show that between 1894 and April 1905, Mary filed more than a dozen birth certificates for illegitimate children born while in her care to young mothers with names like Dora, Emma, Sarah, Lizzie, Rosa, Kate, and Effie. Mary's home—of her own volition—became a haven for these girls and their unwanted babies and for other needy children.

Mary did not hesitate to express her opinion regarding the possible public influences leading to the downfall of these girls.

SPOKANE, Washington, February 23 [1901]—To the Editor of the Spokesman-Review:

A news item in this morning's issue of your paper gives us the not unusual information that some one's wife down in the country had "gone with a handsomer man," or, at any rate, with a man whom she cared for more than the one she had promised to "love and honor till death do us part"—leaving her little boy as well—the greater sin of the two. But the part of this commonplace story that attracted attention most of all was her doubtless true story that going to dances where she met her particeps criminis [Latin for "partner in crime"] was the cause of her downfall. . . .

I feel sure that I can say, without fear of contradiction, that while no sort of dance is calculated to elevate morality, the public dances, and more especially country dances, are more productive of real evil than all of the other social follies of today. Drinking and carousing come afterward.

Public country dances are so much more productive of evil than public city dances because there is most always no restraint—everything goes. . . .

Let me say to the mothers of young girls, and to any one having young girls in their keeping: Keep them away from public balls. I feel sure that in my 13 years of professional life here no one has seen more of the dreadful consequences of this sort of entertainment than myself, and I feel that I know whereof I speak.

I know of at least a score of girls and women whose downfall can be traced directly to the evil influences of midnight dances.
—MARY A. LATHAM

Mary's association with infants and children in the city took many forms. From delivering babies to delivering children to the orphanage, from setting broken bones to breaking the sad news of a death, Mary faced whatever came before her. She went where she was summoned.

"The Baby Will Probably Die" was the headline of a March 21, 1891, article in the *Chronicle*. What followed was a reporter's account of an accident, during which a mother and her eight-month-old baby were thrown from their light buggy after a wheel "went down into the slot in the cable road [roadway with cable inserted for cable cars to run]." The injured infant and mother were taken to a nearby hotel and Mary was summoned. She later reported, "The baby's skull is fractured and there is little hopes [*sic*] of its recovery . . . there is some prospect that the child will get well, but I do not think it probable."

"A Sad, Sad Story" was the next compelling tale in the ever-faithful *Chronicle*. A quite detailed description unfolded of a "prosperous Swede farmer" coming to the Palouse wheat-farming region to scout for a future home, leaving his young wife and two sons behind in the Flathead Valley of Montana. Regrettably, while staying in Spokane the farmer received news from a neighbor that his wife was being unfaithful. After racing back to Montana on horseback to claim his wife and property, he returned to Spokane defeated, his only traveling companion his three-year-old son.

At this point, Mary enters the story: "This morning about 9 o'clock a strongly built, neatly dressed, plain featured Swede entered Mrs. Dr. Latham's office in the Blalock block . . . He said he wanted Mrs. Latham to place his little boy in St. Joseph orphanage." telling her he'd left behind his "faithless wife" and infant son, who would later come to Spokane. He asked Mary to help them as well. "Mrs. Latham kindly consented to place his little boy in the care of the sisters, and to do as he requested when his wife should arrive with the other one." This experience was not a new one for Mary, who was quoted as saying, "That is one case in a thousand similar ones."

On the pages of the *Spokane Review*, in November 1891, "The New School Board" was the headline, followed by "Directors of the Library Association Want Mrs. Latham." William Branch, president of the school board, wrote:

> *To the Patrons and Supporters of the Public Schools of Spokane: as a large proportion of the taxpayers of our city are women, as well as a majority of them teachers, it seems only a matter of justice that at least one member of the board should be a lady; and recognizing the superior natural, as well as educational, qualifications of Dr. Mary A. Latham for this position of trust and honor, we, the directors of the Union Library Association, do hereby recommend her to the support*

and suffrages of all friends of our public schools as a member of the
board of education of this city.

That same month, more letters to the editor supported Mr. Branch's proposition to elect Mary. Someone only identified as "A." wrote in part, "To find a woman capable of filling such a position is not difficult. A woman who can conduct her personal affairs in business life successfully can surely be efficient and helpful on a board of education. If a personal reference is needed I suggest the name of Mrs. Dr. Mary Latham as one fully qualified to fill such a position."

John E. Allen agreed, "If we are to have a lady member of the school board, [a first] by all means, let us have Dr. Mary A. Latham, providing she will accept. There is no one in the county better qualified, and having been a teacher in the public schools in Ohio, knows what is needed in the line of education. Her work for the public library entitles her to the respect of all interested in education."

However, *Mrs.* John E. Allen disagreed in a response letter, saying, "My husband . . . was the first man in this city to suggest the name of Mrs. Latham for the school board, and I, woman like, voted against her. It was because we need her in the sick room and we need her in her newspaper work, for by her ready pen and fearless way of using it she is doing more good than many of the ministers, so we need her in every place except politics."

It is clear that Mary was a natural fit for the position, and yet her name is not mentioned either as an officer or a member of the board of education of 1891, 1893, 1897, or 1900—the only years mentioned in Edwards's *Illustrated History*.

Turning from campaigning for the school board, if indeed she was, to a more basic concern for children, the *Semi-Weekly Spokesman-Review* published "Without a Home" in December 1892. The author attempted to lighten the mood by adding: "An Infant with Troubles Enough to Be Bald-Headed." The story feels like fiction but unfolds as the truth of how one John Klein was arrested for "trying to dispose of a two-weeks-old infant he was carrying in his arms." Apparently, Mary's process of placing foundlings did not always go smoothly.

John Klein was escorted into the Blalock Building and Mary's office, where he offered a dozen different explanations as to why he had this newborn in his possession. The *Spokesman-Review* stated: "He denied that he had been to several variety shows the night before, and that he had tried to induce the girls, inmates of the places, to adopt his infant. His stories were getting more and more bewildering, until finally, with a wrench, he blurted out: 'Dr. Mary Latham knows all about this kid.'"

The story of how Klein came to bring "this kid" to Spokane is complicated. But it did begin with Mary. She explained how some months earlier she had received a letter from a woman in Idaho who had been pregnant, but became ill; the child she was expecting died. She implored Mary to find an infant for her and her husband to adopt. "I have been the means of having several children adopted into reputable families," noted Mary. Soon she received another letter from Lewiston, Idaho, asking her to bring a baby for the woman.

And a third letter arrived, this time from Pullman, Washington. Apparently, not too many days later, according to Mary, "a nice-looking woman came into my office and asked for the baby to take to Pullman. That night we drove 50 miles out into the country and back. It was a stormy night, with the wind blowing and howling, and I never felt better than when I returned safe with the little infant. I had got it from an unfortunate girl. It was born a little over two weeks ago. Her mother consented to the transfer."

While Mary was satisfied she had found a good home for the infant, she was sadly unaware of the young wife's deceit. The glow of a successful placement diminished quickly at the appearance of young Klein, who accused Mary of playing "a pretty trick." He explained that when he returned home, his young wife had presented the infant (the child from the wild buggy ride) to him as their newborn son. The paper described Klein's reaction: "John suspected something. He had some sense, even if he is only 22 years old, and has a head shaped like a sugar loaf. The child was too big and strong to be a newly born infant, and he cross-examined his wife, [who] confessed."

Klein attempted to extort money from Mary for his troubles, in the end asking for only enough money to leave town. Mary steadfastly refused him, suggesting, "I think this is a case for the police, and we might as well call them in." In the face of Mary's rebuff and threat to summon law enforcement, Klein left Spokane.

In closing, the article stated: "In conjunction with the real mother, Dr. Latham will look out for the baby's welfare. It is a beautiful child and the doctor has no fears but that it will soon be adopted by some charitably disposed couple." In fact, in early January, a two-paragraph bit in the *Spokane Review* confirmed it:

> *John Crabb, Jr., is now the name of the three weeks' old infant which John Klein threw back on Dr. Mary Latham's hands a few days ago.*
> . . .
> *The day after the little boy was returned to Dr. Mary Latham, Mr. and Mrs. John Crabb . . . decided to adopt him as their son. Yesterday Judge Moore appointed Dr. Mary Latham legal guardian to the baby, and the necessary papers were signed by her, making Mr. and Mrs. Crabb the adoptive parents of the young one.*

Another of Mary's charitable actions emerged when a young pregnant girl was found wandering the streets and was brought to Mary's office. Mary responded when later interviewed, "I would like to help hang the man who got this poor creature in this trouble." As was par for the course, Mary took in and tended to the girl in her own home. "I think our laws are far too lenient concerning this matter. . . . The most aggravating feature, so far as the girls are concerned, is that to seem blindly in love with the man who cause [*sic*] their trouble, and no matter how stupid or sick, they will shield him with their dying breath. And these heartaches and heartbreaks will go on forever as a result of woman's love and weakness."

A bit of the Old West arrived in Mary's life in March 1897, when the mother of a newborn affected by an extreme case of postpartum blues brandished a pistol. "The matter was brought to the attention of Dr. Mary Latham, who at once visited the distraught woman. Ladies from the Deaconess home cared for Mrs. Stevenson and her baby Friday night, and yesterday they were taken to Dr. Latham's home. Dr. Latham said yesterday that the woman is suffering from puerperal mania, no uncommon trouble under similar conditions, and all that is necessary for her complete recovery is rest and freedom from worry."

If a patient was being threatened, folks knew to watch out for Mary, who was bold in her protection. In the early 1900s, this headline appeared: "Abandoned Babe Dies—Dr. Mary Latham Tells of Girl's Betrayal." Mary had signed the infant's Notice of Death, which brought investigators to her door, filled with questions. Mary did not want to talk, although she finally said, "The mother of the child is a respectable young woman. What her name is or where she came from, if I do know I will not make public property. It is sufficient to say that the child was denied the right to a name, which was the cause of it all." Mary had received a call about the birth, she said, adding, "[W]ho it was is none of your business." The caller had begged Mary to find a home for the illegitimate infant, identified as "a pretty brown-eyed baby girl," but the child had died before Mary even had a chance.

Mary proceeded to explain to the investigators—the past educator in her probably eager to enlighten and perhaps boast a bit—that "This sort of thing is not uncommon. I have heard of many instances such as this, of young women coming to the city from the country or smaller towns to hide their shame. I have found homes for more than one hundred children who have been deserted, or their parents were unable to care for them," she said, her words revealing her pride. "I was a member of the first home-finding society ever founded in Spokane, twenty years ago."

Not all was sadness and drama for Mary. One pleasant-sounding event may have been a favorite of hers. In September 1897 there was to be a

"Baby Show" as entertainment at the regional fruit fair. "A happy selection of competent judges has been made by Dr. Mary Latham . . . [And] not only the Fairfield [a small farming town thirty miles southeast] quadruplets, but also triplets and twins" were scheduled to be at the show for all to see, noted the *Spokane Chronicle*.

The Baby Show evolved into a Babies Day in 1899, sure to have provided pure enjoyment for Mary. The *Chronicle* quaintly informed its readers: "There will be a baby show at the Spokane industrial exposition . . . All that remains is for the fond mammas to dress their 'little tootsie-wootsies' in their best and take them before the committee on the day chosen." The paper reminded folks that Mary was the manager of Babies Day and, given that she had been away in Alaska the previous year, it was imperative they hold the event now that she was back. The paper included information about prize donations: "Mayor Comstock and Dr. Mary Latham have already given silver cups." Citizens came forward to donate an assortment of other prizes.

Following the event, a further lengthy description filled a column on the front page of the *Chronicle* and flowed into subsequent pages, painting a thorough picture of the happy day. Headlined "Seventy Plump and Pretty Babies Smiled and Cooed and Squalled," the article noted that "Eight of the prettiest prize babies and two pairs of twins are being shown to admiring friends today by the 10 proudest mammas who ever entered their infants in a prize competition. . . . The success of the baby show is due in a large measure to Dr. Mary A. Latham."

Several homes for unwed mothers existed within the city, and one came to Mary's attention. She had a personal connection to this home, and naturally, she published her thoughts.

SPOKANE, Washington, October 9 [1902]—To the Editor of the Chronicle:

Referring to the recent esclandre [French for an incident that arouses unpleasant talk or gives rise to scandal] anent [Scottish for concerning] the Florence Crittenton Home. I feel impelled to say that

Matron Eichholtz is strictly right in the position she has taken, and that the consensus of opinion of the conservative community is with her. While I have never been directly interested in the Crittenton home I have always been interested in the class of girls called unfortunate, and when the home was established was delighted, feeling that a long felt want was about to be filled, and proved my faith by sending the first four girls who were inmates. Imagine my astonishment and disgust, when in a most appealing letter, smuggled to me by one of them, I was informed that no matter how sick or blue, or what the conditions might be, each one had to open her door to visitors to be stared at like so many "dumb driven cattle" on exhibition to the morbid curious sightseer, as if the burden of the poor creatures were not already heavy enough.

After that you can well believe my interest in the institution flagged, and I have found other places in which my poor girls could be cared for. . . .

I believe that Matron Eichholtz can not be excelled in her ability to manage a place such as that was intended to be, and the fact that the majority of inmates followed her in her exodus proves that they trust her, and trust in those cases is more than all beside.
—MARY A. LATHAM, MD

One Jno. M. Palmer, disturbed by the noise and enthusiasm emanating from the Salvation Army band in the streets of Spokane, wrote a letter to the editor:

Dr. Mary Latham, whose kind heart and ready pen are always on the right side, has succeeded in having the little [unfortunate] girls kept from marching with Salvation Army folks; the chief of police has abated the drum nuisance; the army is forbidden to march on Howard street; now is there not some way by which the whole of the racket could be silenced, or at any rate can they be corralled in the place where they belong and be made to stay there until they can behave like people?

The Salvation Army has been voted a nuisance in many places, and should be here, though all are ready to [g]ive the devil his due, and admit that the leaders in the movement here are not [a] bad sort of people.

CHAPTER 10

For a Public Library

SPOKANE, Washington, July 1 [1891]—To the Editor of the Chronicle:

Let no one think for a moment that there is any dissention in the ranks of the Union Library association, for there is none, they are just working right on, adding new books and interesting features daily, and hoping as a result of the entertainment to be given to-night at the Presbyterian church, to be able to add many new books to the already large collection.

While we dislike more than we can say, that there should be any newspaper notoriety . . . you know that sometimes the "uses of adversity are sweet," and that these seeming disasters often ultimate[ly] [result] in good.

Hoping the public will interest themselves in these matters sufficiently to learn the truth, and that they will feel as I and as anyone else interested feels, that is, that there cannot be too many good books no matter in whose possession they maybe, [sic] if the public can use them.

I remain, very truly,

—MARY A. LATHAM

This letter of Mary's seemed to be in response to another and seemed to be addressing negative comments from the community. Then someone wrote again: "We can not [*sic*] have too many book[s]—i.e., good books—and it is only the croak of the pessimist, who, like the poor, are with us always—who says the book business is overdone, etc." The tone of the letter, signed only "M.," seems reminiscent of Mary's voice.

In an October issue of the *Review*, Mary's letter to the editor started with a question: "What has become of the public library movement?" Mary favored "a consolidation of the small private libraries which she had helped to establish and the unions' reading room." In her letter, Mary urged people to get behind the campaign to create a public library, "for surely there can be none who are uninterested." Mary argues for the library, stating, "Our children, in whom the craving for knowledge is innate, can then be learning some thing [*sic*] good, or at any rate can never remain ignorant for the lack of opportunity for learning."

Mary had been campaigning for a public library since first arriving in Spokane Falls, although the Great Fire of 1889 had interrupted her crusade. "[T]he fire," wrote Mary, "had made us all such heavy losers that nothing had been done lately, the struggle for bread and butter having been in many cases the all-absorbing subject for consideration. But it seems to me that our hardest times are now over." She went on to promise that as soon as the proposed library was a certainty, she would donate a set of the *Encyclopedia Britannica*. Mary was promising to put her money where her mind was.

On November 16, 1890, a brief article in the *Spokane Falls Review*—without a byline—again urged citizens to support the plan for a library. "No city is truly great where wealth and pleasure reign supreme. Spokane Falls needs a public library. It would be better to dispense with parks than with a storehouse of the world's wisdom."

Almost daily and into the next year, Spokanites were listening to and reading about the concept of a library that would be open to all citizens. A successful fundraiser was held in June of 1891. Speakers were listed inside its program, including "Essay—Dr. Mary A. Latham." It was reported that "Mrs. Latham's essay . . . was a picturesque and unusually original effort, and was very pleasantly received." The entire essay was printed in the newspaper, with a covering comment, "Dr. Latham's Scalpel: It Cuts a Certain Class of Aristocracy to the Quick." Mary had done just that, reading her essay to the crowd, urging the audience to come together and to examine their lives for what was most important. In a descriptive paragraph, detailing all kinds of people who might come together, and for what reasons, she said in part, "Some came . . . hoping thereby to erase from memory's page a chapter of dark disgrace—an accursed spot that would not out." How strangely prophetic these words became for the unsuspecting Mary.

In early 1893, Mary was still working the cause. The *Review* again mentions Mary, announcing that "L. Baldwin and Dr. Mary Latham were elected trustees [of the Union Library Association] for the ensuing term." The name "L. Baldwin" would appear twelve years later during one of the worst days of Mary's life—the signature below a statement demonstrating compassion.

January 1894 brought another report regarding a meeting of the labor unions to elect a new librarian. At the end of the article, which listed various unions—plumbers, miners, printers, cigar makers, tailors, tinners, to name several—was a list of new delegates, including Mary's son, Warren Latham, from the plumbers' union, and "Dr. Mary A. Latham and Eugene Bertrand from the honorary members."

Mary's active support of libraries was lifelong. Serving on the Spokane library's board of directors, she helped to canvass neighborhoods for book donations. By 1904, she was still serving, this time on the committee for the purchase of books. In September of that year, a crowning achievement for Mary, her fellow library supporters, and the entire community came to fruition, when construction began on a Carnegie library, built with money donated by Scottish American businessman and philanthropist Andrew Carnegie, who was responsible for libraries being built across the nation.

CHAPTER 11

Pity the Poor Farm

SPOKANE, Washington, June 2 [1892]—To the Editor of the Review:

> *Today I received a letter from a former patient of mine, a most worthy woman, who, through a series of misfortunes, including ill-health, has been driven to seek shelter in the poor farm at Spangle. She speaks of being in every way comfortable, of the very great kindness of the physician there, and winds up by saying that the idle time hangs most heavily upon the patients, and asks that if possible I could send them something to read. Now I would like to ask some of the readers of The Review to send occasionally a book or a magazine or novel to these unfortunates, or send them to me and I will forward them, and thus assist some of "the least of these" to while away a few of the many weary hours which fate has willed should be spent in a way which, as in the case of the one of whom I speak, is more bitter than death.*
> *—MARY A. LATHAM*

In the year 1892, the poor farm was in trouble. In June the *Spokane Review* reported at length under the column heading, "Poor Farm Investigation." It began: "One of the prominent members of the Ladies' Benevolent Society yesterday informed a *Review* reporter that a delegation from their body would attend the investigation into the condition of the poor farm at Spangle . . . to see fair play [done]."

Six society members' names were posted at the bottom of the report, which included the following disturbing scenario: "At the farm we found the superintendent thereof abundantly supplied with all the necessaries and conveniences to make the place comfortable and to insure its cleanliness, but notwithstanding this it was the poorest kept, most squalid looking and withal the filthiest institution we ever saw." Perhaps sensitive to how this statement might affect the manager, the ladies added the following: "We [reported] the condition in which we found the institution, which was in regard to the dirt of the place, not how it was managed."

In the year following that investigation, Superintendent Dawson from the poor farm wrote to Mary to thank her for a donation of books at Christmastime. As 1895 dawned, a new superintendent had been appointed, according to the *Chronicle*: "Wm. Pittam . . . has been appointed superintendent of the poor farm at Spangle in the place of R. W. Butler." Mr. Butler had been sent to take charge of the poor farm in Whitman County. In the span of just two years, three superintendents had managed the Spangle establishment. Pittam later writes to Mary to thank her for a box of books sent for the benefit of the residents.

Honoring her word to her former patient, Mary continued her campaign to provide reading material for residents, reminding the citizens of Spokane in the paper with headlines like "Will Cheer the Poor," and "Who Has Magazines?"

In 1903, the county poor farm, described as "more of a hospital for the needy and indigent," was still a farm that spread across 160 acres, all of which were cultivated and planted, making the institution self-sufficient. Each of the inmates—as lodgers were called—had a job to do, whether it was milking cows, splitting firewood, or tending gardens. Wheat also was grown to use as barter for merchandise or food that could not be grown.

Men who lived at the poor farm were reported to make an annual exodus from the place during the spring, in order to find wage-earning work on farms or with the railroad.

In 1914, a new infirmary was constructed on the site of the poor farm, which may have interested Mary. It was reported that "a special Northern Pacific train will carry citizens and county officials to the institution"—an important service for the county. This was also the year World War I broke out in Europe following the assassination of Archduke Franz Ferdinand.

The new infirmary would serve as a place for injured soldiers to convalesce. During the war years, groups of inmates waited on the platform of the farm's railroad siding for each expected train in order to gather any papers left behind carrying news of the war. The train crew handed them over to the men, who carried them back to be distributed among the inmates.

The *Spokesman-Review* of August 29, 1915, gave a detailed report of the farm:

Spokane's version of a county "poorhouse" is a brick and concrete thoroughly modern building of three stories set back in a wide green lawn into which the orchard overflows. . . . The farm includes 240 acres of good land, all of which is in cultivation. It is a first-class property, operated on the theory that if the mission it is designed to serve is worth serving at all it is worth serving well. . . . It will be there, a secure and comfortable haven for human wreckage, through numerous generations. That is the idea Spokane has undertaken to exemplify in the new county infirmary, substantial and sanitary assurance that those who need care will receive the best that can [be] given with the means available.

In the year before Mary's death, and two years after Prohibition had been declared, a significant change was noted regarding the poor farm. The *Spokane Chronicle* shared statistics: "Under prohibition there has been a steady decrease in the number of persons at the county poor farm at Spangle." More than once Mary had proclaimed that she was not a prohibitionist. Perchance this article caused her to pause and reconsider her stand on the issue.

CHAPTER 12

End of a Marriage

SPOKANE, Washington, Semi-Weekly Spokesman-Review, March 13, 1900: "Marriage and Divorce," by Mary A. Latham of Spokane, awarded second prize in the second series of editorials by women:

Does it never occur to those who are constantly finding fault . . . that if the laws relative to the granting of marriage licenses made it more difficult to secure a permit to enter matrimony that the necessity for divorce laws would be almost nil?

A few years ago the ministerial union of this city, after days of deliberation and argument pro and con, framed a set of resolutions to be sent to the legislature asking that body to limit the grounds on which divorce could be obtained. This, most reverend sirs, was beginning at the wrong end. Let your resolutions be that the issuance of marriage licenses should be so restricted that no one unable to give a history of a sound mind in a sound body, a good moral character and a visible means to support a family should be allowed to marry.

Better still, let the sacredness of marriage vows be instilled into the minds of children, or at least as soon as they enter young man and womanhood. . . . Young people rush headlong into matrimony, giving never a thought to the sacredness of the vow—"For better or for worse, till death do us part," and are rarely instructed by older and wiser heads that to marry for social position, for wealth, for a home, aye, for anything save love and affection, brings everything but the happiness hoped for . . .

We quote the following from a well-known writer [probably Mary's sister Eliza] on the above subjects: "Ministers are keen enough *to join in marriage all sorts and conditions of men and women and pocket their fees for it, but when it comes to divorce they throw all the blame on somebody else. . . .*

"They are willing to unite drunkards, gamblers, epileptics, thieves, immoral characters and all diseased persons fast enough. They will join a worn out roue [sic] whose life has been one round of immorality, to the sweetest, purest girl in Christendom, and call it God's holy ordinance. Shame on such priests!

"Let the preachers who are so ready to perform these marriage ceremonies look to themselves and their responsibility for the prevalence of divorce."

Sound and logical, is it not?
—MARY A. LATHAM, MD

By the time Mary wrote her editorial about marriage and divorce, she had experienced both with Edward.

When he'd finally arrived in Spokane Falls during 1889 and joined her practice in the prestigious Frankfurt Block, Mary was already well recognized as an important newcomer. Was it premonitory that on August 4, 1889, only five days after Edward's arrival, most of downtown Spokane Falls—including the Latham office and home—would be consumed in a voracious runaway fire?

Seven months after the fire, the *Spokane Falls Review* of March 11, 1890, announced that Edward and Mary's "Office and dispensary [are on the] southwest corner of Stevens and Sprague. Residence on the Island." This has to mean Havermale Island, which must be where they found refuge after their fresh hopes, plans, and dreams went up in smoke. In due time, their marriage appeared to have turned to ashes as well, with Edward moving nearly as far north as possible without entering the country of Canada.

It appears that Mary traveled north at least once to see Edward. An article in August of 1892 announced, "Mrs. Dr. Latham . . . will spend the remaining part of the summer with her husband, Dr. E. H. Latham." Perhaps this was a last attempt at keeping the marriage together. Two years later, Edward sued Mary for divorce, stating abandonment from the time she had left Ohio.

Then, on July 19, 1895, came this statement: "A decree was signed yesterday by Judge Arthur granting to E. H. Latham an absolute divorce from Mary A. Latham."

━ ⌣ ━

Edward's assignment to Colville was first mentioned in the *Seattle Post-Intelligencer* in December 1890: "Dr. E. H. Latham of Spokane Falls was today recommended to be physician at . . . Colville reservation." There he reportedly found satisfaction in what would become his life's work. When not caring for patients, Edward spent much of his time using photography to capture thoughtful and historically valuable images on the reservation. In fact, in 1981, fifty-three years after his death, fifteen of his photographs were displayed inside the Oregon governor's office. Although Edward found a great deal of enjoyment through his photography work, he would meet incredible challenges through his medical station, where he lived in a small home built for one.

Soon after Edward arrived in Nespelem to serve the reservation tribes, influenza arrived as well, fiercely attacking the populace. A headline in the April 1891 issue of the *Butte Weekly Miner*—in extremely poor taste but indicative of the time—announced, "Heap Bad Cold." "*La Grippe* [French for influenza] is rapidly thinning the ranks of the Spokane tribe of Indians and Nespelem Indians on the Colville reservation. About 500 are down with the malady and many are dying. Dr. E. H. Latham of Spokane . . . thought he had conquered the disease, or at least had it under control, but now it has broken out worse than ever before, so that the doctor is detained indefinitely on the reservation."

The following year, Edward filed his "Report of Physician at Colville Agency." He had much to report regarding the several tribes he served, which he described as "Okanagans," the "Nespelims," the "Sanpuell Indians," "Moses' Band of Columbins," "Joseph's Band of Nez Percés," the "Colville and Lake tribes," and the "Lower Spokanes." In his extremely thorough report, Edward detailed each tribe's religious practice, living conditions, moral and sanitary conditions, and each tribe's attitude toward him.

The road to building good doctor–patient relationships among the tribes was rocky. Edward needed to prove his skill. Especially proud of his relationship with the Nespelem, he stated, "I have succeeded in gaining their confidence . . . To use their own language, I am their 'tillicum,' which means the same as brother." Of Chief Moses Edward said, "Old Chief Moses is very much of a gentleman." Of the Lower Spokanes, he could "only speak with praise. They are all Christians, belonging to the Presbyterian Church."

After reporting at length on each tribe, Edward all but begged the government to send at least one other physician to help him, reminding the powers that be: "In all this vast reservation there is no hospital of any kind. . . . One is needed very badly."

To end his report, he shared that nine births had transpired, adding, "The Indian women are very superstitious . . . and would die before they would submit to a white doctor attending them in confinement." And: "I must say that the medicines sent are not in all cases what I would wish." He closes with, "I am, very respectfully, E. H. Latham, Agency Physician, Nespelim [sic], Colville Reservation."

Chief Joseph had been one of Edward's patients. Following Joseph's death in 1904, Edward is quoted by the Evening Statesman of Walla Walla, Washington, as saying the oft-heard line, "Chief Joseph died of a broken heart." Edward added, "Grief was all that ailed him. In vain I tried to console him." While talking about Chief Joseph having been removed from the Wallowa Mountains region of the Northwest, Edward was reported to have said, "From that time Joseph was never the same man. He brooded constantly over the fact that Wallowa, the country of his youth and of his dreams, was going farther and farther from him, and that the region about his new home at Nespelem was year by year growing smaller and smaller through the encroachment of the prospector and the settler. In recent months this grief has resulted in a bent form, in a listliss [sic] life, which ended in death." He described how at "the grave of Joseph, a bell will wave on a tall, slender pole of hemlock. Its tinkle will make peace with the spirits of the dead, according to an ancient Indian legend."

Five years passed after the death of Chief Joseph with no newsworthy event being reported from Colville. Then, in 1909, word reached the newspapers that Edward was dealing with another serious situation. "An epidemic of smallpox," the report began, "is sweeping over the south half of the Colville Indian reservation, and strict orders have been issued . . . [by] Dr. E. H. Latham to ferrymen forbidding them [from] either carrying the Indians off the reservation or the whites on."

Some thought Edward was not fulfilling the duties of his position. There had been statements that he was drinking too much and "press rumors about the doctor's competence." An Indian Agent, former army captain John McAdam Webster, sent a "staff efficiency report" in 1909 regarding Edward:

> *[Latham] is a superannuated gentleman who has not kept up with his profession, and has vegetated and hibernated at Nespelem for the past 18 years; is kindly, hospitable and charitable; has accumulated enough money to buy a nice place on Lake Chelan, which has increased in value since he purchased it. He has exhibited more energy in the past, but is too old and indolent to be efficient, and I rate him "Fair."*

Edward retired the following year.

—◆—

The news of Edward's divorce suit against Mary had traveled fast, reaching Ohio, where the *Cincinnati Enquirer* presented the doleful story on July 26, 1895, under the bold title: "Doctors Fell Out. They Were Husband and Wife, and Are Separated." The article shared "information from the Far West. Word has been received in this city that E. H. Latham, an old resident of Columbus, has been granted an absolute divorce from Mary A. Latham, at Spokane, Washington." The column praised Edward, reminding readers that he was the son of the late Belle (sometimes spelled *Bela*) Latham who had been postmaster of Columbus for nearly twenty years; that his brother, Milton B. Latham, came to represent California in the United States Senate; and that the Latham family "was among the oldest settlers of Columbus." The only mention of Mary was that she was "a well-known practicing physician."

Mary had not been afraid to say she was unhappy with the divorce suit, of course. In 1896, *The Woman's Medical Journal* carried an article written by Mary and previously published by a Spokane newspaper, the *Outburst*. Expressing her strong views against divorce being granted in the courts for "insufficient reasons," her view was not the ordinary idea of the day.

Next, the *Spokane Chronicle* published a letter to the editor: "Don't Let Them Marry. Dr. Mary Latham Would Forbid Blessing and Banns." While responding to an article entitled, "Shall the Divorce Laws Be Revised?" Mary tackled this subject with aplomb in her award-winning essay, "Marriage and Divorce."

"I cannot refrain," she began, "from saying that marriage licenses are too easily obtained, and our officers should see to it, as far as in their power lay, that no improper persons should be allowed a license, and our common law relating to this matter should allow no cripple, no habitual drunkard, no one of unsound mind, no one addicted to the cocaine, morphine or kindred habits, no one addicted to the divorce habit . . . to marry."

By today's standards this sounds like a harsh statement, and politically incorrect. However, this statement of her beliefs regarding the issue must certainly have been driven by her experience of placing for adoption so many abandoned babies and children, by the experience of delivering malformed infants, and by her own unwelcomed divorce. Mary finished by quoting a writer (probably her sister Eliza) from "a New York paper": "If all of the criminals and other improper people were prevented from marriage, the criminal and divorce lawyers could go fishing."

There's no way to know whether James, twenty-five, and Warren, twenty-four, now students living in the college town of Walla Walla, read Mary's published letters. On January 24, 1896, the *Spokane Chronicle* observed: "Dr. Mary A. Latham left for Walla Walla this morning to visit her sons, who are attending college there. She expects to remain until Sunday." Neither she nor her sons could have known that ten years later, nearly to the day, Mary would return to Walla Walla, facing a prison sentence.

CHAPTER 13

The Isabellas

SPOKANE FALLS, Washington, January 22 [1890]—To the Editor of the Review:

In a recently received letter, Matilda Joslyn Gage [a respected suffragist] urges me to interview personally the "liberal minded, intelligent women of our city" in regard to the—to her mind—all-important subject of the ballot for women.

The task she has imposed upon me is Herculean. The name of the "liberal minded, intelligent women" in Spokane Falls "is legion—for they are many." I am equally sure that all such are not for indiscriminate suffrage for women. There are many women here who, like myself, believe that the liberty of the ballot should be based not on the accident of sex, money, "previous condition," or in fact anything except the broad plane of intelligence (the sine qua non [Latin for "without which there is nothing"] of all good), and that a simple-minded or uneducated woman has no more business with the ballot than a baboon, or even a drunken ward politician.

I can not think that the coming of the milliernnium [sic] will be on the day when the law for woman suffrage is passed, or that any sudden radical change will be produced by the passage of such a law, but that social, moral and political purity will come only by drawing a line so finely that neither a mental nor a moral imbecile of either sex can use the ballot.

Press of business prevents my compliance with Mrs. Gage's request, but I trust that some of the ladies of our city . . . will be able to

assist those good ladies who have devoted their lives, money and influ-
ence to benefit their sex.
   —MARY A. LATHAM

In New Zealand even the splendid big native Maori women vote.
   —ELIZA ARCHARD CONNER

In 1893, Mary "was elected Chairman of the Medical Department of the Washington Branch of the Queen Isabella Association and in that role represented the State of Washington at the Chicago World's Fair Columbian Exposition," according to Gidley. The fair was planned to commemorate "the Quadro-Centennial of Columbus' discovery of the New World," as explained by author Lauren Alexander Maxwell in her honors thesis, "Constructions of Femininity: Women and the World's Columbian Exposition."

The Queen Isabella Association (QIA) was made up primarily of women doctors and lawyers who supported women's suffrage and equal rights. Its members wanted to compete with men on an equal basis. The Isabellas, as they were called, hoped to erect a statue at the fair of Queen Isabella of Castile, "acknowledging her as the 'codiscoverer of the New World,'" according to Maxwell.

Before the fair even opened its gates in 1893, a conflict arose between the QIA and the Board of Lady Managers (BLM) regarding how women ought to be represented at the exposition. The BLM was a government agency, and its Spokane branch was led by another early influencer, Alice Ide Houghton. Seeking only general reform for women, not equal rights, the Lady Managers believed women ought to be most exalted inside the home.

Led in Chicago by its president, Bertha Palmer, the BLM were, informed Maxwell, "more concerned with the expansion of women's roles as mothers and wives into the public realm than with fighting for both political and social equality with men."

Because of this conflict, the Isabellas would not join in the Woman's Building at the fair where the BLM were located. Members of the QIA were likely to be women who sought higher education in order to reach goals of work that would support and fulfill them into old age. That idea, along with striving for suffrage and equal rights, placed the Isabellas in a category of women "considered abnormal by society at large." Mary certainly fit this category, having earned the label of *abnormal* while earning her medical diploma in 1886. And as if that were not enough, she moved without her husband to the far-flung Washington Territory.

There was much discussion between the two groups and the Exposition Committee leading up to the fair, which included a refusal from the construction committee to the QIA's request to build their own pavilion. The Isabellas didn't accept this, but instead began campaigning for private investors. The QIA successfully funded the construction of their own pavilion several blocks from the fairground. Mary could have been a contributor. Or, if indeed she attended the fair as stated by Gidley, she was likely involved in all stages of creating the pavilion.

The World's Columbian Exposition, exclaimed one reporter for the *Evening Telegraph* of Bucyrus, Ohio, "has been made the occasion and the scene for the assembling of a series of remarkable and notable gatherings of the trained and cultivated experimenters and thinkers among the nations of the earth."

Many of those "experimenters and thinkers" entered the hall nicknamed the "Isabella club house," which was built adjoining the Isabella Hotel. The building was mentioned in many reports as the location of a number of events, including, "The world fair congress of women physicians." An article in the *Brooklyn Daily Eagle* said, "Some months ago there was organized an association of women physicians, surgeons and trained nurses to take charge of an emergency hospital during the exposition. Eastern women do not begin yet to appreciate the great work done by these enthusiastic western women." More groups were mentioned: "The first meeting of women lawyers ever [was] held [there.] . . . Members of the Non-Partisan Woman's Christian Temperance Union . . . [and] both the art and musical departments of the Queen Isabella Association [were there.]"

May 1893, the first month of the fair, was a much-touted success. No doubt members of the QIA would have shown interest in one particularly transformative event. The *Seattle Post-Intelligencer* described what had surely been a strong draw for certain women.

> *There were lively times today in . . . meetings . . . of the woman's congress being in session in the great art palace on the lake front. . . . Mrs. May Wright Sewall[,] . . . president of the International Council of Women, presided over the department on dress reform. She appeared in a reform costume, with a full skirt cut eighteen inches from the floor, and her limbs below the border were encased in neat-fitting blue leggings.*

This striking new fashion was enthusiastically received by women in the audience.

Perhaps even more enthusiastically received was the appearance of Susan B. Anthony, who climbed to the podium and "read a paper prepared by Elizabeth Cady Stanton on civil and social evolution of women."

Susan B. Anthony was lauded by Mary's sister, Eliza, who was said to have "associated with" both Anthony and Stanton. In 1907, she wrote, "Susan B. Anthony was so loyal to her own sex that she never employed a man in any professional or industrial capacity if she could get a woman to perform the service she wanted. She never gave an item to a man reporter if she could find a woman reporter."

There was at least one female on the editorial staff of the *Spokesman-Review* for the years 1910 to 1913, named Bertha Grether. Because of what is known of Mary's support of women, it's likely she—like Anthony—would have sought a woman employee and may have worked with Grether.

—◦—

Tragically, on July 10, calamity struck the World's Fair. A large cold storage warehouse inside the exhibition grounds burned. Twenty-three Chicago firemen died fighting the blaze. After the fire, the executive committee for the Exposition resolved that all receipts received for the following

Sunday admission would "be used in aid of the sufferers who sacrificed themselves while performing their duty."

Excepting the tragic fire, the World's Fair of 1893 was deemed a success, especially considering that 1893 was the first of four years the United States was affected by the financial Panic of 1893. Unnumbered Americans were left financially shaken or ruined. Financial uncertainty could be one explanation why Mary may not have attended the World's Columbian Exposition. However, she likely fulfilled her responsibility of promoting the Exposition locally.

CHAPTER 14

Klondike Fever!

Spokane Chronicle: "The Klondike Craze—A Syndicate of Women are Arranging to Go Next Spring"—

Klondike mania has attacked the women, says the New York Press. They have it in violent form. Wealthy business women, writers, servants, all sorts and conditions of women, seem to have fallen victims to this particular form of financial disease. . . .

The New York contingent has arranged its expedition . . . under the title of "Woman's Expedition to the Klondike Gold Fields. To be known as the Woman's Klondike Syndicate." . . .

The expedition will be personally conducted by Mrs. Sarah W. McDannold, a member of the International League of Press Clubs, and of the State Federation of Women's clubs . . . Mrs. Eliza Archard Connor, authoress and member of the Women's Press club, is vice-president.

Mrs. McDannold described the event for the reporter:

The object of our expedition is to prospect and locate mining claims on the Klondike and other tributaries of the Yukon river, to establish a new mining camp and hospitals, and to equip a complete commissariat train. Within the last three days fifty nurses have asked to go with us, and, while we need but one physician on this trip, a dozen have applied. . . .

We will leave New York on March 1, and it is a six months' trip. The officers——Miss Boswell, Mrs. Connor and Mrs. Pierce—and I will go. My son and Mrs. Connor's also, will remain there.

The editor of the paper added this bracketed comment below the article: "[The Mrs. E. A. Connor . . . is a sister of Dr. Mary Latham of this city, and it is more than possible the doctor will arrange to accompany the expedition.]"

———

Fourth of July at Unalaska, Aleutian Island, Alaska [July 22, 1898]—To the Editor of the Chronicle:

We have been lying here at anchor for a fortnight, and a quieter existence could not be imagined up to the morning of the Fourth, when at the striking of eight bells we were roused by the booming of cannon, the snapping of pistols and the etcetera of the celebration of Independence Day. . . .

If half of the stories are to be believed, this northwest is a veritable Eldorado . . . the new strike at St. Michaels [sic] is the richest of all, and several men have gold to show in proof of what they say . . . I would say "Better stay away," or "be sure of something before you start."

—MARY A. LATHAM

A respite was due Mary from her demanding work. One came in the shape of a steamer pass worth $300 [more than $9,800 today]. It read: "To the Captain of the Steamer *Santuit*: Pass Dr. Mary Latham from Seattle to Dawson City. Wm. C. Gates, Pres't T. T. & M. Co." The *Spokane Chronicle* shared the exciting news: "Scattering Klondike Gold. How Swiftwater Bill Remembered a Spokane Friend." Details were given: "A free trip to Alaska; a block of stock in a big Klondike company; cold cash to settle all debts booked against him or his relatives—hundreds of dollars of it; and the promise of a $10,000 [more than $328,000 today] hospital to be built in Spokane, Seattle, Dawson City, anywhere she chooses—that is the way the Klondike gold king paid his debts to Dr. Mary Latham when he passed through Spokane."

Mary clarified why Gates was generous:

It was away back in the days just after the fire . . . [O]ne day there came a call to go out to Shantytown to see a boy named Will Gates, who was down with the typhoid. I found young Gates in a little shack in Shantytown—a black-haired youth of twenty years or so, who had the fever sure enough. He was a very sick boy, but we pulled him through; and he seemed so grateful that we didn't feel bad even if he couldn't square up the bill after he got well.

The reporter asked Mary, "Are you going to Alaska?"

"Yes," she replied. "In May I shall close my offices and store everything and go to Alaska for a visit."

<hr>

Soon, "Dr. Latham Has Gone," was the headline on June 16, 1898. The article revealed: "A letter has been received from Dr. Mary A. Latham. Dr. Latham has been in San Francisco for the past week or two. It is probable she will go to the Klondike before returning to Spokane before fall. The present trip is for the benefit of her health and a summer vacation. She is traveling with the family of her brother-in-law." *Family of her brother-in-law* seems like an odd turn of phrase. Who were they?

<hr>

Even artists and entertainers were infected with "Klondike fever." Published in full shortly before Mary set sail for Alaska, this ballad is a clever advertisement for the city of Spokane, as evidenced in the first stanza:

There's many thousand people rushing madly to the field,
Away up north where mother earth, her golden grains doth yield.
The whole world on one errand bent, the rich and poor alike,
Are northward bound, and all will try, to reach the rich Klondike.
They are coming from the east, from the south and from the west,
All striving hard to get there by the way that seems the best.
Now I call their attention to the latest news that's out,
It gives the tip to Argonauts to take the Spokane route.

Mary had a significant issue to consider before leaving: her application for a patent on a homestead near the settlement of Marshall, which was eight miles south-southwest of Spokane. She would need permission from the government to take a leave of absence because her travel dates would fall within her homestead "proving-up" period. After contacting authorities, she was granted permission; they would put her proving-up period on hold.

———

Before leaving, Mary agreed to report to the *Spokane Chronicle*. On July 7, her first dispatch arrived from Dutch Harbor, Unalaska, of the Aleutian Islands.

Her words reflect her state of restfulness. Mary enclosed three specimens of local flowers with her first update, identifying one as a violet. She further described: "The climate is lovely and we wear no heavier clothing here than in Spokane." Her boat was anchored in Dutch Harbor, she said, having sailed for ten days from San Francisco with a "cloudless sky and almost waveless sea." It seems Mary either did not redeem Gates's Seattle steamer pass, or it was applied to the longer route. Steamboats, she reported, were being prepared to take her and others up the Yukon River to Dawson City.

But while visiting Dutch Harbor, Mary met Mrs. J. Stanley Brown, daughter of President Garfield, whom she described as "a very sweet-faced woman with whom it is a pleasure to converse." Quite taken by the settlement, Mary described her surroundings: "Jersey Cows, fat, meek-eyed and gentle," roamed close by; there was "a lovely little lake" from which Dutch Harbor took its water supply; "a mammoth Plymouth Rock chanticleer" who woke them every morning with his crowing; "a bumble-bees' nest on a side hill"; and "a pansy bed" plump with color.

Closing her report with a prediction, she wrote, "Should the output of gold from the north continue (and there is abundant prospect of it if half the stories be true) a city will spring up in this place and it will become a fashionable place to spend the summer." Just before her byline, Mary added, "After one has spent half a life in work this lazy manner of living is for the time at least the acme of happiness. Will write again from St. Michaels [*sic*]."

MISSION OF THE HOLY CROSS, ALASKA, July 20 [1898]—
To the Editor of the Chronicle:
We are now 500 miles up the Yukon, having left St. Michaels [sic]
four days ago, and have made little progress . . . But our trip so far has
been one of almost unalloyed delight, and there would be no regrets of
any sort were not the summer season here so short. . . . Many and var-
ied were the sights, and long were the days in which to see. Once, after
our 6 o'clock dinner, our party went on the upper deck to see the sun
set and rise, all of which was accomplished in less than two hours . . .
Surely, if any people on earth need the influence of civilization
they are these filthy creatures whose very origin seems a myth, and
whose manner of life resembles that of the animals rather than the
human . . . At this mission the people are now growing potatoes, cab-
bage and all ordinary vegetables; also berries, while the hills are cov-
ered with wild roses and other flowers. . . . [And there is] delightfully
green grass, reminding one of the Palouse wheatfields [sic] in May."
. . . I must not forget to mention the raspberries, the currants, blueber-
ries and "salmon" berries . . . the currants especially being large, juicy
and just what a Spokane housekeeper would like for jelly.
—MARY A. LATHAM

It was August when Mary reported from Dawson City on the banks of the Yukon River, where she would spend ten days. Situated at the center of the Klondike Gold Rush, both geographically and chronologically; the Gold Rush radiated from Dawson City during the years 1896 to 1899. Her report was published on September 17, 1898: "The house I live in is a 5-room log and board one, good and substantial, and the property of Mrs. Anna Minehan, formerly of Spokane." Mary described the house, surrounded closely by tents occupied by men, noting that she and Anna couldn't help but overhear their conversations.

When Mary shared her reaction to witnessing two funeral processions in one day, it was a harsh reminder of the perils of the Klondike gold-prospecting life. The processions, followed by men carrying spades over their shoulders, were carrying caskets of people who had died from typhoid fever. Mary affirmed the scene: "And what wonder! There is no disguising the fact that this is the dirtiest city in Christendom . . . The heat is something terrific and the odors from the slimy streets and dirty meat shops are full of death." Saddened, she wrote how one funeral party was "leaving somebody's boy asleep in the icy mould [*sic*] three feet deep." Little did she know that within five years she would share that devastating experience.

Her report included religious and medical scenes: "Close by is a Catholic church. . . ." And, describing what was likely of particular interest to her: "There are two hospitals here, one Catholic and one Episcopalian, both of which are ever crowded." Surely this wasn't just hearsay, as it's very likely Mary would have visited both hospitals.

In spite of the frequent deaths and the "perpetual daylight" that she described as "a very unpleasant feature of life here," Mary reveled in her period of rejuvenation in the North. Perhaps she was partly invigorated by camaraderie, as several other Spokanites were there. Mary provided an informative list of professional men who were in Dawson City: "Colonels

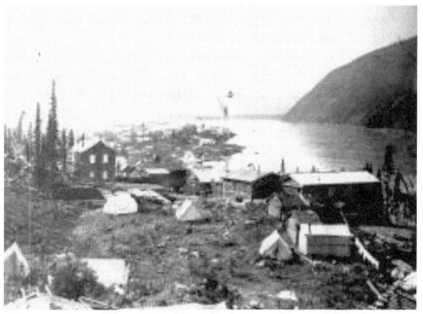

Photo showing Dawson City in 1898, looking south toward hospital buildings.
PHOTOGRAPH BY ERIC A. HEGG / PUBLIC DOMAIN

O. V. Davis and O. D. Garrison, both of whom like Dawson; Drs. New-man and Bruner . . . the former will start home soon; Mr. Newkirk . . . has made a fine stake and is going to Europe this winter; Mr. Wilson who had the La Belle restaurant in the Frankfort [Frankfurt] block . . . and Populist Foster, who will go with Dr. Newman; Gus Seiffert is in business here." She added the names of two women: "Mrs. Humphreys and Mrs. Holgate are now over here, lately from Skagway."

━━ ⌣ ━━

Mary does not mention the presence of her sister, Eliza. Yet, in the June 24, 1899, issue of the *Fort Wayne* [Indiana] *Evening Sentinel*, is this arti-cle: "Plucky Woman War Correspondent: Eliza Archard Conner, Who Is Carrying a Typewriter Around the World," by Bessie Dow Bates. Bates was reporting about Eliza when she wrote about the 1899–1902 Philippine-American War. But she included this: "Some 15 months ago she started for the Klondike." Calculating from the article's date of pub-lication, it should have been March or April of 1898 when Eliza started for the Klondike. This concurs with the previous article quoting Mrs. McDannold, who stated that the Alaska-bound New York entourage, including Eliza, would leave New York on March 1. Since Mary "left [San Francisco] on the 11th [of June] . . . for Sitka, Alaska," and did not return home until October, the likelihood they were in Alaska at the same time is strong.

"From Dawson City," Bates added about Eliza, "she sent a series of correspondence articles which were widely printed." It appears the sisters were in Dawson City at the same time.

Months before Eliza left New York for the Klondike, an article appeared in the *Akron Beacon Journal*: "Two missionaries," it said, "were last August sent to the Klondike by two New York women under the auspices of the Presbyterian board of home missions. The names of the women are kept a secret by the board." Could one of the women have been Eliza? Her father, James Archard, had been active in the Presbyte-rian church in Ohio. It's reasonable to think Eliza might have visited a Presbyterian church in New York City, if she walked through the doors of any church, being a believer in reincarnation. Regardless, now she was

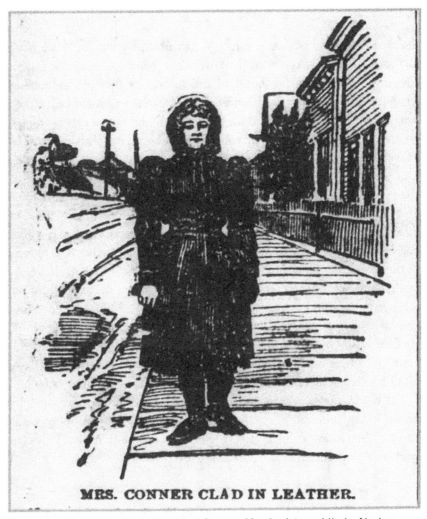

MRS. CONNER CLAD IN LEATHER.

Newspaper depiction of Eliza Archard Conner, Mary's sister, while in Alaska.
COURTESY OF HARRISBURG TELEGRAPH [PENNSYLVANIA], AUGUST 30, 1898, NEWSPAPERS.COM

traveling to Alaska and the same region as the missionaries, who had reported they "started a Young People's Society of Christian Endeavor and a branch of the Y.M.C.A." And: "I walked over 20 miles on Tuesday with the thermometer at 37 degrees below zero, made 11 calls and found about 30 church people who will attend the meetings."

The *Beacon Journal* received more reports from the Klondike. "The Rush to the Klondike is Assuming Notable Proportions," one article began, advising that between five hundred and six hundred people had already left New York City for the Klondike. One citizen was Rene Lepreux, "a druggist, who has been located for some time in the Yukon region and has established stores at Skagguay [*sic*] and Dawson City." This is someone Mary likely sought out since her son, Frank, was a druggist.

The "King of the Klondike" was Alexander McDonald, "Big Alex" to most. The *Marion* (Ohio) *Star* in September 1898 reported that Big Alex had been in the Klondike for the previous two years, making him present in the region the same time as Mary. He was noted as "one of the newly made plutocrats of the Klondike." And yet, like many miners, he did not come from wealth. He had "scraped together about $400 . . . went to his employer and resigned." Then pointing his face toward the Alaska Gold Rush region, he arrived filled with determination. "The success of his clean up [retrieving every bit of gold from sluice boxes] this year has made him literally a fetich [archaic spelling of 'fetish,' likely meaning 'icon']."

It would not be surprising if Mary met Big Alex in Dawson City, knowing her admiration for hardworking people who made good. In addition, she knew W. C. Gates, who was, according to Mary, Alexander McDonald's partner.

What a wild—in every sense of the word—experience this must have been for the fifty-four-year-old physician and woman of conscience from the State of Washington. The nation—indeed, the world—was fascinated by what was happening in Alaska and the Yukon. The State Department in Washington, DC, received a communication in 1898 "from the United States Consul at Dawson City. In it he says that Dawson City is built upon a bog, and has a population of 20,000 . . . Lots on Main street cost $40,000 [more than $1,300,000 today]."

Money was important to Mary, but probably of more value while in the Klondike was her acquaintance with Swiftwater Bill. Mr. Gates, as the respectable Mary called him, had offered to build her a hospital in Dawson City in recognition of Mary saving his life. Would Mary accept his offer? Would Gates follow through?

And what kind of offer had Swiftwater Bill made to James, Mary's son? According to a notice in the *Spokane Chronicle* in April 1898, titled "Called to Alaska": "A telegram was received yesterday by Dr. Mary Latham from 'Swiftwater Bill' Gates notifying her that Gates' steamer would sail from Seattle tomorrow." Gates asked Mary to ask James to make haste to Seattle to catch the steamer. The article explained that while Gates was in Spokane, James had accepted "an excellent offer," and that he would "proceed at once to Dawson City via the river route." As a journeyman plumber, it's feasible that James went to Alaska to ply his trade for Swiftwater Bill. But James was also invested in mines near home, so perhaps he went for the gold.

Plenty of records remain concerning Swiftwater Bill Gates, including several derogatory articles with headlines like "Gates Under Arrest," "Women Demand Money," "Swiftwater Tells Court He's 'Broke,'" "Bill Gates Declares He Is a Bankrupt," "Swiftwater Asks for the Legal Beggars' Allowance," "Gates Asks for Son: Court Refuses Plea," "Old Swiftwater Gets into More Hot Water," and finally, "Swiftwater Bill Caused Trouble."

Mary had read enough, and she said so in the September 17, 1898, issue of the *Chronicle*:

W. C. Gates, "Swiftwater Bill," is making more money than ever and is going out soon on his way to London with Alex McDonald, the richest man in Klondike, whose partner he is. Just why the newspapers take such savage delight in printing all those ridiculous stories about Mr. Gates is hard to say, as he is one of the foremost business men in Dawson and well respected. A prominent business man said to me concerning him: "Almost all the stories printed about 'Bill' are outrageous falsehoods, the outcome of jealousy, and as for me I'd rather take Bill's word than some of their notes. He is just the kind of a man we need in Dawson."

Mary ended her article with a bit of nostalgia. "Dawson City is a great place, the only one of its kind in the world. But there is another and a greater, namely, Spokane, also the only one of its kind, and as Washington holds all that is near and dear to me, I feel a home longing I cannot resist."

Her home longing may have been fortuitous, since typhoid fever was spreading like wildfire, thinning the ranks of the gold seekers. As reported by the *Cincinnati Enquirer* around the time Mary began to travel south, "many old timers have been stricken with the scourge . . . [It is] estimated . . . [at] not less than 3,000 case[s] of typhoid fever." Even if Mary had felt the call to administer care to the vast numbers of sufferers, there would have been little one doctor could have done.

—◦—

From Dawson City another Spokane woman returned home, Miss Anna Moyer. Early in October 1898 she offered observations from her travels, and one included Mary: "Dr. Mary Latham left Dawson City about the same time I did, but she went by the St. Michael route, and probably will not be here for two or three weeks yet. Her trip to the Klondike was simply to look at the country, but she says she is going back in the spring to start a drug store."

It's important to mention that at about this time, the name of Mary's sister, Letitia—or Mrs. L. A. Buckley—appeared in the *Spokesman-Review*: "Mrs. L. A. Buckley of Cincinnati is in the city on a visit to her daughter, Mrs. Philip Richmond. She will await here the return from the Klondike of her sister, Mrs. Eliza Archard Conner, the New York journalist, who is in Dawson City in the interest of the American Press Association." Oddly, there's no mention of Mary joining the reunion of sisters. Probably happy to be in Spokane, Letitia could not have known that within two years, she would receive an urgent plea to return.

—◦—

On October 24, 1898, the *Chronicle* reprinted a *Seattle Times* piece, whose reporter had interviewed the popular Mary Latham upon her return to Seattle aboard the steamship SS *Roanoke*. The article, which identified

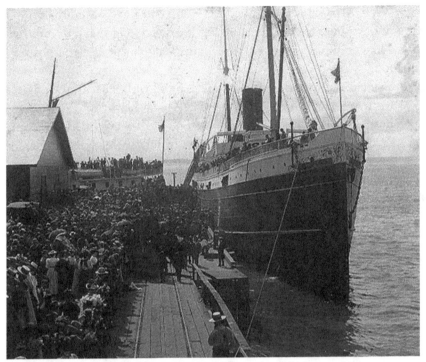

The *Roanoke*, the steamer on which Mary returned to Seattle in 1898.
PHOTOGRAPH BY FRANK LA ROCHE / PUBLIC DOMAIN

Mary as having "traveled extensively in Mexico as well as in Alaska and the Yukon territory," spent most of the column space sharing Mary's advice on "the best way to carry dresses." Two years before, a brief article reported that Mary had traveled to Los Angeles, returning through San Francisco and Portland, Oregon. Apparently, during her travels, Mary had perfected the art of packing.

Mary arrived home safely and in a satisfied state of mind. In an article headlined "Swiftwater Kept His Word," the *Chronicle* reported that Mary was now "the only woman in Washington who has been from the mouth of the Yukon river to the lakes which form its source."

She was also asked about Swiftwater Bill.

"Well, Mr. Gates made good his word, and I can have my hospital at any time; but [I] have been taking it easy so long that I do not feel at all like going to work just now. I am going to the Paris Exposition in 1900."

Coincidentally, perhaps, there was to be a World's Medical Congress in Paris that same summer. Mary added, "[I] may not go into active practice until after that." Mary did deliver one illegitimate child in February 1900 to an eighteen-year-old mother. In July, she delivered an infant for the wife of a soldier. Another half-dozen Mary-assisted deliveries occurred in the fall of 1900.

But Paris in 1900? What about her homestead near Marshall, and the five-year occupancy and proving-up law? Her health no longer a concern, Mary needed to focus on her homestead. The reporter asked, "You do not regret your trip [to Alaska] in any way?"

"On the contrary," Mary said. "I am repaid a thousand times, having better health than [I've had] for years. I have seen the great northwest in its aboriginal state and would not have missed the trip for anything."

The eyes of the world left the goldfields of the Klondike and traveled to Europe, where Mary planned to attend what everyone was talking about: the Paris Exposition, as briefly described in an article entitled: "Exposition Universelle (1900)."

April 14, 1900
Gates opened to the World Fair, the Great Exposition in Paris. For a few months 210 temporary pavilions from different countries and architectural styles lined the Seine. The Exposition Universale [sic] included the Exposition Decennale [sic], an art show of painting and sculpture from the previous decade. The first working escalator was manufactured by the Otis Elevator Company for the Paris Exposition. During the expo Rudolf Diesel demonstrated an engine that ran on peanut oil.

While it's certain that Mary's sister, Eliza, was in Paris for the Exposition, it's not known whether Mary managed to go. Given her proclivity to write about her travels and with no reports found, it seems a reasonable deduction that she did not make it to the Exposition.

Eliza—no doubt striding about the fairgrounds, even at sixty-two years of age, with her curious mind abuzz, pad and pen in her pocket— wrote "Paris and Her Show," on March 24, 1900. This article was preliminary to opening day, written somewhat like a tourist guide of what to expect. On May 7, she wrote about the day she "spent in the grounds to see what was what," commenting, "[I]t is pretty, and it is Paris out and out." Reporting about her experience, not all of which was positive, she claimed the World's Columbian Exposition of 1893 in Chicago had been much more expansive than this one, although she did remark that "Paris is architecturally the grandest and most beautiful city of the earth. It did not impress me so much . . . 18 years ago . . . but then I was homesick and miserable and had not yet learned to be at home wherever fate flings me."

Eliza's name appeared in a Paris-related column in the *Chicago Tribune*, headlined "Editors in Council: Ideas Concerning the Destiny of Modern Newspapers." A lengthy deck followed:

> *Bulky Sunday Journals Discussed and Their Doom Prophesied—Influence of "Patent Insides" on the Individuality of Provincial Weeklies— Editing Papers with a Saw and Scissors—Speech by an Enthusiastic Woman Who Reports Horse Races and Baseball Games.*

A list of speakers for the program of the day included this: Address— "The Evolution of the Newspaper Woman," Mrs. Eliza Archard Conner, New York City.

———

Perhaps Mary decided to forgo her Paris dream, choosing instead to be conscientious about her potential land grant. Obliged to honor the Homestead Act, passed in the 37th Congress in 1862, she would have read the declaration: "That any person who is the head of a family . . . and is a citizen of the United States . . . [is] entitled to enter one quarter section . . . and that said entry is made for the purpose of actual settlement and cultivation . . . That no certificate shall be given or patent issued therefore until the expiration of five years from the date of such entry . . ."

Another possibility is that Mary may have planned all along to avail herself of Section 8 of the Homestead Act: "*And be it further enacted,* That nothing in this act shall be so construed as to prevent any person . . . from paying the minimum price, or the price to which the same may have graduated, for the quantity of land so entered . . ."

From the moment she left Ohio, Mary had intended to purchase land in the West. And she had followed through with her intention by purchasing real estate in the area. Deed records show that in November of 1889, Mary purchased a city lot in the South Park Addition to Spokane Falls for $450 (more than $13,000 today). A few years later, she bought acreage located in "Section 14, township 24, range 42E" in Spokane County. This was a quarter-section of land (160 acres) situated several miles south between Spokane and the Marshall Junction of the railroad, near Hangman Creek. For this land, Mary completed a homestead application, on which she noted that she developed plans for a ranch, described as "[making] valuable improvements . . . consisting of a house worth $100, a barn worth $75, a $10 chicken house and . . . [to plant] 7 acres to rye."

Eighty-eight separate deed records of properties were found showing Mary A. Latham and/or James or Warren as either grantor or grantee.

Six months into her Marshall ranch project, everything came to a halt. Mary explained: "I located the 120 acres January 11, 1898, for the purpose of a homestead and made the necessary improvements till June 11, when my health failed . . . I got a leave of absence from the authorities at Washington [DC] from June 11, 1898, till June 11, 1899, and went to Alaska." Mary swears on the affidavit applying for leave of absence that "she is in ill health, being troubled with chronic nervous prostration, and that it is necessary in order to recover her health that she take a change of climate."

Now she was back, but upon returning to the homestead, she learned someone else had been studying the Homestead Act, especially Section 5:

And it be further enacted, *That if, at any time after the filing of the affidavit . . . and before the expiration of the five years aforesaid, it*

shall be proven after due notice to the settler, to the satisfaction of the
register of the land office, that the person having filed such affidavit
shall have actually changed his or her residence or abandoned the said
land for more than six months at any time, then and in that event the
land so entered shall revert to the government.

There arose a disagreement, and it very nearly started with a bang. On June 17, 1899, the *Spokesman-Review* reported the following: "Information was filed last evening in the superior court against Loren C. Fenn (sometimes spelled Penn) charging him with assault with a deadly weapon. Fenn is the man who drew a gun on Dr. Mary A. Latham during a dispute over some land at Marshall. He will be arraigned before Judge Prather this morning."

In August, another paper celebrated, stating: "Dr. Latham is a Winner. . . . She Can Keep Her Homestead Says Register Ludden. Dr. Mary Latham has won her land contest, which has been in the United States land office for the past three months."

Fenn had come to Mary's office, she said, soon after she returned from her travels, stating "that he was a poor man with a family . . . that if I would let him stay on the place to take care of it till my leave of absence ran out it would help him out. I thought I was doing a good deed and gave him the permission, thinking it would be all right." Now Fenn had unsuccessfully claimed, along with witnesses he brought, that Mary had not been seen on the land. Mary explained that she was "in the city all day attending to her practice and spent the nights at the ranch." The land in question, through which Marshall Creek flowed and railroad tracks traveled to the depot east of town, was quite desirable.

Fenn scoffed at the idea that Mary had received her leave of absence "on the plea that she was ill." Because Mary traveled to the Klondike—as was previously well documented in local newspapers—Fenn insisted this fact "ought to prove that she was as well as any woman." His point of view is perhaps understandable. Still, Mary had been granted the leave of absence, protecting her right to the land.

Three years passed, when, like an iceberg bobbing to the surface, news about Mary and Alaska appeared. The topic was luggage. A large trunk, which had been left behind in Alaska by Mary—thinking she would soon return—had arrived in Spokane. As an aside, the article added that she had "secured several lots at the townsite [*sic*] of Eagle City."

Eagle City was founded by dissatisfied gold diggers prospecting the Canadian side of the Yukon and paying taxes to Canada on their gold. Frustration at the heavy taxation drove them across the border, where they decided to "survey for a townsite at a bend in the river not far from where Athabascan Han Indians had a camp called David's Village." This was the same place where the Hudson Bay Company had once run a trading post. Covetous of more settlers, these founders sent an agent to Dawson City to "throw the newly-platted lots on the market where they were 'readily sold at good figures.'" One account stated that those buying lots drew slips of paper from a hat to choose which lot was theirs. It's easy to imagine Mary's face, her excitement contained, when the hat came before her.

The validity of these transactions was questioned later that year in the *Klondike Nugget*, with suggestions of a "peculiar proposition" and "a big scheme." Nevertheless, Eagle City may have been where Mary hoped to return when she came north again.

Despite her hopes and well-laid plans, she would never return.

This begs more than one question: Did Mary simply abandon those lots? Did she sell them for a handsome profit? Was it a bogus transaction? The answers are unknown. What was known were the contents of the trunk, which were "curios rare and interesting . . . some specimens of the moss on which the reindeer feed, some rare shells from the beach on Norton's bay, Indian relics, footwear, walrus teeth and many other curiosities."

Mary's aim had been to return and spend a winter in the frozen North. But, in less than two years, her life would change so dramatically that this dream and many of her other aspirations would forever remain unfulfilled.

CHAPTER 15

From Helpful to Harried

The editor's patronizing heading: "Dr. Mary Latham Writes a Cute Letter about Law and Lawyers":
SPOKANE, Washington, January 15 [1894]—To the Editor of the Chronicle:

> *In regard to the vapory mouthings, [sic] meaningless hints, threats of arrest of various women who are taking an interest in the Marie Neilson case, the whole affair is a ridiculous joke and not worth minding, save it is making some of the ladies a trifle nervous. When Marie Neilson came to me on Saturday, weary, tearful and almost sick, begging me to do something to prevent the proposed examination, I said nothing to her, but to her friends I said: "There is no law in heaven or on earth to compel a sane, virtuous woman to submit to such an ordeal against her wishes." . . . Others have expressed themselves in a like manner. I distinctly remember hearing Judge Arthur say a few months ago: "Law is a very simple proposition—the embodiment of common sense."*
>
> *[T]he women . . . are only carrying out their convictions for conscience sake. All this reminds me of hearing some ladies in conversation. Said one: "But you know the devil himself was said to be a lawyer at one time." Said the other: "Yes, but the women outwitted him."*
> *—MARY LATHAM*

The subject of Mary's January 1894 letter to the editor at the *Chronicle* was a court case wherein one Marie Neilson (also spelled Nielson), a housemaid, had claimed "an assault upon her person," by her employer,

Herman Lawrence [————]. A charge of rape was filed with the superior court. One article by an observer inside the courtroom described how Marie "was present, heavily veiled and surrounded by women." Neilson was likely surrounded by members of the Women's (sometimes Woman's) Health Protective Association, an active group formed after the original association was founded in New York City the previous decade.

The protective actions of the women would prove unnecessary that day because court was canceled. The young woman was promptly ordered to be gynecologically examined by "a commission of doctors." In fact, it appears Neilson was to present her body for pelvic examination to a group of six men: Dr. N. Fred Essig, a member of the Washington State Board of Health; Dr. C. S. Penfield, secretary of the Washington State Medical Examining Board; Dr. Byrne, an alumnus of the Northwestern University Medical School (Chicago Medical College); Dr. Alexander MacLeod, an immigrant from Nova Scotia who settled in Spangle; Dr. G. D. Russell, one of the handful of physicians who began practicing in Spokane in 1887, and in whose office the examination was to take place; and Dr. D. L. Smith, president of the Free Coinage Republican Club in the city.

"Mrs. Dr. Latham promised to produce the girl," noted the *Chronicle*, "and later notified the commission that she was not in a condition to be examined." Another detail in a different article stated: "About twenty ladies appeared with Miss Neilson shortly after, but the girl refused to be examined."

Then came an ominous statement: "It was claimed yesterday afternoon that several persons had conspired to defeat the purpose of the courts, and it was stated that they would be brought up for contempt." Mary quickly advised that she had not prevented nor conspired to prevent Marie Neilson from reporting to the commission of doctors for examination:

Miss Neilson came to me [and] gave good reasons why the examination should not take place and requested me to prevent it if possible. I ascertained that her story was true and telephoned as much to Dr. Russell. When I received word that all the doctors were waiting, Miss Neilson and her companion left my office and I have not seen them since. . . .

I am not, as many suppose, a member of the Woman's Protective Association, but I am willing to help whenever I can in a good cause. I sincerely hope that these women will be all the name of their society implies. As for the threats of the attorneys for the defense, I do not dread them for I have done nothing that would make me unwilling to submit to arrest for contempt of court. If I should be convinced that the defense is in the right, I shall be just as willing to assist that side. I have been dragged into the whole affair most unwillingly.

In the following day's paper, another letter confirmed her stand.

SPOKANE, Washington, January 16 [1894]—To the Editor of the Chronicle:
I desire, through the columns of your paper, to thank the two score or more of people—whose friendship is most to be desired—who have manifested their good will and approval of my course in the Marie Nielson case by calling, writing, or by telephone messages. While the subject is up, I wish to say that I have never attended a meeting of the W.P.A. [Women's Protective Association], have never gone purposely from my office in the matter, and my every interview with the girl was when she came to my office. My interest in this affair has been from a humanitarian standpoint, and to make less heavy the almost overwhelming burdens of a most unfortunate young woman. And had she been my daughter, or sister, or even my servant girl, I should (knowing what I do about this most atrocious affair) have resisted to the utmost the examination of yesterday, as, in her condition, the additional unnecessary torture entailed upon her thereby, would have the effect of an additional assault. Besides nothing worth while [sic] could be gained by so doing.
   —MARY A. LATHAM

How fortunate the women of Spokane were to have a standard-bearer such as Mary. A benefit to help Neilson was organized and notification posted. The announcement offered details for the upcoming program, to be held in the Music Hall, including this: "Professor John Welin will give a tightwire and juggling exhibition, and Dr. Ehrnholm will perform several feats of legerdemain [conjuring tricks with one's hands]. Dancing will follow." How astonishing this kind of support must have seemed to a humble housemaid going up against a well-known businessman.

—◆—

At the time, Mary's future looked bright and bountiful. She was well respected for the reputation she had so laboriously earned.

Yet, about a year later clouds rolled in as the Mix Nursery Company opened a case suing Mary for $2,800 (more than $91,000 today), according to the *Semi-Weekly Spokesman-Review* of January 1895. An agreement had been signed between Mary and Mix Nursery Company of Moscow, Idaho, and one S. J. Genoways of Spokane, to "furnish and plant . . . two thousand apple trees; one thousand standard pear; two hundred cherry trees; two thousand prunes; four thousand grape vine; five thousand black berries; ten thousand raspberries." This was an extraordinary undertaking, yet Mary approached the task with enthusiasm—or was it naiveté?

The Mix Nursery Company was under contract to care for all that was planted "on land subsequently conveyed by Mrs. Latham to H. Warner." Mix Nursery complained the conveyance was actually without consideration and therefore the land was still owned by Mary, leaving her financially responsible. Could the conveyance have been a stall tactic, an attempt to buy time to find a monetary solution? The nursery claimed she owed $500 (more than $16,000 today) in damages and requested enforcement of a lien upon her land.

By April, this action had come to be known as "the fruit tree case." Mary claimed the nursery stock she'd been sold was no good, and she aimed to prove it in the most convincing way. With a touch of chutzpah, Mary had some of those very trees brought into the courtroom as evidence of her claim. The newspaper declared: "Quick and inanimate fruit trees . . . in all stages of growth and decline, adorned the equity courtroom yesterday as silent witnesses in the suit of the Mix Nursery Company against Mary A. Latham."

In the end, despite being surrounded by her army of trees, Mary did not win her battle against the nursery company. A judgment of $1,279 (more than $41,000 today) was secured against her. With that, her more serious pecuniary troubles began.

⌐ ⌐

By the spring of 1897, Mary pushed back, turning the tables inside the courtroom to sue one of Spokane's most prominent citizens, Colonel William Ridpath. "Suit has been commenced," announced the *Semi-Weekly Spokesman-Review*, "by Attorneys Jones, Voorhees & Stephens in the name of Mrs. Mary Latham against W. M. Ridpath for possession of 200 shares of Le Roi mining stock." The Le Roi was a copper and gold mine in British Columbia, owned by a group known as the Spokane Colonels, including Ridpath. As evidence of his obligation, Mary presented an instrument bearing the following statement: "Due Mrs. Mary Latham two hundred shares of Le Roy min'g. stock. [Signed] W. M. RIDPATH."

"Upon this showing," the article continued, "the plaintiff prays judgment that the defendant be required to transfer to her 200 shares of the Le Roi Mining and Smelting Company's stock." Otherwise, she expected to be paid the equivalent value. It's interesting to find that Daniel W. Henley, who was a vice president of the Le Roi Mining and Smelting Company, would serve as Mary's defense lawyer in 1905.

⌐ ⌐

Another year, another lawsuit.

It was 1901 and Mary was at the courthouse, having been sued along with one Henry L. Earnest. Attorneys A. E. Barnes and George A. Latimer were bringing the suit. Apparently, Earnest had been charged with "larceny by embezzlement." What was Mary doing in the company of a supposed embezzler? Perhaps Mary trusted others too readily. A December 1901 article in the *Chronicle* advised that Barnes and Latimer had requested an order for money to be deposited in the court registry. The attorneys claimed that "money was wrongfully withdrawn by Mary A. Latham at the order of Henry J. Earnest, and upon the representations of Charles P. Lund and L. R. Hamblen, attorneys."

Surrounded by a band of men who appeared to be advising her, could she have been so gullible as to associate with an embezzler? It may be that the plaintiffs, attorneys themselves, chose to use the harshest of terms in order to make a point.

⌒⌒

Despite her troubles in court, Mary carried on. For example, in May 1901, it was announced that "the *Western Woman's Home Magazine* . . . is expected to come from the press in this city about June 1. The publisher and editor will be Dr. Mary A. Latham, who has had considerable experience as a writer. It is to appear once a month in neat magazine form and will be planned to especially interest the women of the west."

Another record states that she published a novel titled *The Witch's Wreath*. While no copy was located, one could speculate that the plot might center around a German folkloric superstition that claims witches cause feathers in a bed to weave themselves into a wreath, and that whoever sleeps on it will become ill, dying when the ends of the wreath come together.

No matter the plot of her novel, Mary remained a prolific writer of letters to editors, essays, short stories, and articles, often for the benefit of women, but always speaking with a woman's mind—her own.

⌒⌒

Mary's continuing saga included a clever headline in 1902: "Editors Have Troubles Too." The ownership of the *Stevens County Reveille* of Colville was now in question. Though a Stevens County affair, most of the litigants lived in Spokane County; Mary among them. In an almost vaudevillian-style tale, the reporter explains that Rufus H. Wood had been sole owner of the *Reveille*, and that

> *Wood later sold the other half of the paper to G. S. Wilson, who still owns that interest. Wood used his $525 note as collateral security and borrowed $102.40 of J. M. Nelson. Nelson then in turn, it is claimed, sold the note to Mary A. Latham, Dr. Latham selling it to Earnest, and Earnest having made the note and it now having come back into his possession it is alleged the note was satisfied and canceled.*

Was there deceit involved in this tangled web of transactions? Could this have been a carefully orchestrated financial sleight of hand? Was this a con perpetrated by a group of cronies, to which wealthy Mary had been granted membership? If so, was she aware of any wrongdoing, or could she have been an innocent though intelligent, overly trusting—if stubborn—woman caught in a spider's web of deceit spun by a group of wily men?

CHAPTER 16

Tragedy on the Tracks

SPOKANE, Washington, September 25 [1902]—To the Editor of the Chronicle:

Referring to the subject of keeping respectable theaters open on Sunday and the objections made thereto, it seems to me very much like "straining at a gnat and swallowing a camel," as Biblical writ has it. In point of fact, in many respects at least, the legitimate drama is one of the greatest educators in the world and there can be nothing degrading or calculated to lower the standard of morals in even the most puritanical idea thereof, while comedy, with vulgality [sic] eliminated, as is always the case in first class houses, does nothing more than produce laughter, thus waking up the "solar plexus" of which you hear so much nowadays, followed by good digestion and good humor.

The saying, none the less true, though trite, that anything good enough for Monday is good enough for Sunday, brings up the question now warmly discussed in religious circles, whether the first of the seventh day of the week is the "Sabbath of the Lord," but my idea of a Sabbath is this: A man or woman can work for seven days in a week, and if he or she take three or four hours out of 24 for reflection and devotion, that is all the Sabbath they need . . . Of course, I shall not expect all to agree with me in this.

[Y]oung and old, seem to crave divertisment [sic] elsewhere, and they must and will have it, and if they must and will have it on the only day in the week they can call their own, why not give them a chance to see a good play in a reputable house rather than . . . in a disreputable place, one of which, accompanied by my son [likely James],

I visited recently to satisfy myself on one point, vis., that they were running in violation of ordinance 30, section 1, which says no person or persons shall carry on business of any sort [on Sundays] except undertakers, druggists and liverystable [sic] men, in the city of Spokane Falls. . . .

[W]hy not permit a respectable playhouse to open for two or three hours on Sunday . . . [I]t gives respectable workingmen and women a chance which they would otherwise be deprived of, that of seeing good clean dramas in a place they are not ashamed to visit.
—DR. MARY A. LATHAM

Changing the "blue laws" (Sunday-closing laws) was the subject of Mary's latest letter to the editor. Blue laws were regulations that originated in Connecticut in 1781, created to "enforce religious standards, particularly the observance of Sunday as a day of worship or rest, and a restriction on Sunday shopping and activities." Having been originally printed using blue paper, the simple identifier stuck.

It's not surprising that Mary had adopted another cause, being now divorced from Edward and with sons Frank and Warren married. Her relationship with middle son, James, who lived with her, was of prime importance. They seemed to enjoy being together, as evidenced in the letter to the editor above. Sadly, unbeknownst to both of them, there remained only seven months in which to enjoy each other's company.

Perhaps James had tired of the particular demands of being a journeyman plumber, as he had recently taken a well-paying, stable job as a brakeman with the railroad, in the train hub of the Inland Northwest. Little did he know that his employment with Northern Pacific Railway would become the death of him—literally—on April 20, 1903. Two days after his father's fifty-ninth birthday, James was crushed between two railcars he was uncoupling at the crossing of Division Street and Sprague Avenue.

On the morning following the grisly accident, the *Spokane Chronicle* cited these details: "Death was instantaneous and was caused by the crushing of the victim's head between the bumpers." Two days later, the *Spokesman-Review* was more explicit, beginning with the headline: "Train

Runs Over Brakeman." It stated the facts: "While crossing the tracks he was struck, apparently from behind, and knocked down and instantly killed. His head was crushed in and his left hand cut off." Oddly, following this detailed recounting, the reporter revealed that his father, Edward, was in the city and had "made the boy a present of a watch."

These accounts concerning their son's gruesome death must have been torturous for Mary and Edward to read, if indeed they did so. Even more dreadful must have been what Mary, who had been immediately summoned, probably inspected at the morgue—the mangled body of her son. It could be that the physician in her insisted she view his body, while the mother in her must have dreaded facing what she was about to see. Granted, as a physician she had likely witnessed horrible disfigurations before, but this was *her* boy. Since arriving at the village of Spokane Falls, Mary had answered the call to help others. Now, suffering from a pain of this magnitude, there could be no real help for Mary, save for sharing her grief with Edward. She would not even have support from her mother, for Jane Archard had died the year before.

James Latham had been well-liked in the community. He had pursued aspirations. His name was included in an 1898 listing of journeyman plumbers. Chosen to act as marshal for the plumbers' union section of Spokane's Labor Day Parade, this means that if James had gone to Alaska when summoned by Swiftwater Bill, he would have returned to Spokane by September. James continued in the plumbing trade until the year before he died. Because of this, the plumbers' union chose to honor him, and stated so in the press two days after he was killed. At a special meeting, union members adopted him back into the union. Following that action, the union banner was draped at union headquarters in his honor. Members of the plumbers' union sent flowers to the funeral home, where many members attended the funeral service "from Smith's undertaking parlors" in remembrance of James.

—◦—

A tempest of emotions must have swirled in Mary's brain as she attempted to accept the cruel fact of her son's sudden and horrid death. The subsequent physical strain became so great that Mary suffered a stroke, and what followed was a noticeable decline in her critical faculties. She was starting to lose touch with reality, or perhaps she was creating her own more bearable version.

But reality was waiting outside her doorstep, and often what she met there was not pleasant. Any observant person could see the slackening of Mary's spirit, the dulling of her mind, the horrible confusion she was experiencing. Still, others who had much to gain in opposition to her—grieving mother or not—met her in court.

Following James's death, Mary began to show a decided lack of discernment. "Dr. Mary A. Latham," an article began, "boasted this morning that she had turned in more certificates of illegitimate births to the board of health as legitimate than any other physician in the city." Why Mary would reveal (even boast, if true) this fact is beyond comprehension, and it's unknown what preceded such a declaration.

But she went on to brag—or, to set the record straight—that, in fact, Jennie H. Johnston (usually spelled Johnson) gave birth to a child on April 10, 1898, at E1024 Gordon Avenue, the address of Mary's clinic for women. James was living with Mary at that address. Mary had completed and filed a birth certificate categorizing the male child of Johnson as "legitimate" and provided a father's name, age, occupation, and resident state. (It's interesting that she used the first name of "James" for the fictitious father.)

The infant died five days later, and Mary completed the death certificate giving the cause as "valvular heart disease." The death also occurred at the Gordon Avenue address.

Five years later, young Jennie H. Johnson would reenter Mary's life in a most upsetting way.

Mary's final point in what could be called a confession was "that she made the birth legitimate because her son happened to fall in love with the girl-mother while she was at [Mary's] house."

But marriage was not to be for James and Jennie, or for James and any woman. He was buried at the Greenwood Memorial Terrace in Spokane beneath a now-stately spruce tree.

Fifteen years later, his mother would be buried in the plot to the north of James's, which she has shared with his father since Edward's death in 1928.

CHAPTER 17

Make Her Pay

I expect to spend between $20,000 and $25,000 [more than $775,000 today] in the various enterprises . . . I have two saws at work in my mill and have 250,000 feet of timber ready for the saw, and lots more growing on my section of land. My lieutenant is J. M. Nelson, formerly justice of the peace at Colville. He is an expert gardener and farmer. Although he is more than 80 years old, he is a hustler.
—*DR. MARY LATHAM, Spokesman-Review,*
September 27, 1903

The paper further stated: "Her plans include the construction and operation of a large trout hatchery, the storing and sale of spring water ice, the incubation of all kinds of fowl by electrical heat, the operation of electrically heated green houses, where vegetables and flowers will be grown, the diversion of Peone creek to form a fall 30 feet high, which will furnish power to operate an electric plant, and a few other industries . . ."

⁓

In J. M. Nelson, Mary seemed to have found someone to partially fill the void left when James died. Still, 1904 was a trying year for Mary. Though he was gone and buried, James's name would appear frequently during the two years following his death.

By February 1904 the Barnard Manufacturing Company was suing Perry Bartlett, Mary A. Latham, and E. A. Sherwood "to recover $511.53 [more than $15,000 today] and costs" in connection with a note given to the manufacturing company by Mr. Bartlett. This claim must have been related to a contract between James Latham and Perry Bartlett—signed nineteen days before James was killed—whereby James "sells to [Bartlett] all the Saw timber located on the South one-half of [Mead Section 3] at the rate of One Dollar and Twenty-Five cents for each one thousand feet of said timber." Barnard Manufacturing was attempting "to foreclose a chattel mortgage on a quantity of logs and lumber, in which the other defendants claim some interest."

The most convoluted lawsuit and resulting trial came just a year after the dreadful death of James. Mary appeared in court to prove what she must have felt was the most important issue of her life. Struggling to retain ownership of property in Mead, she may have panicked.

The Jennie Johnson whom Mary had delivered of an illegitimate child now claimed to have been engaged to James at the time of his death, and insisted James had willed the property in Mead, along with all of his estate, to her. She filed a complaint to this effect with Spokane County Court in July 1904. Interestingly, "Dr. John Doe Mesner" (John H. Messner, a veterinarian) was also named a defendant, but the case essentially became a "she said, she said" affair.

Johnson asserted that Mary knew it was James's intention to will her his property, and that she (Mary) was hiding the original will "to defraud [Johnson] of her rights." By this time, Mary had given notice that she had "removed [her] office and residence to Mead, Wash. Office at drug store. Patients taken care of."

Mary was a good steward of the Latham land, which had been purchased by James from Northern Pacific Railway on October 13, 1902, for the consideration of $190.73 [more than $6,000 today]. The deed was lengthy and detailed, excluding ownership of a strip of land through which the rail tracks ran. The railroad company also claimed exclusive mineral rights to the land.

Yet, on March 13, 1903, Mary was allowed a Notice of Water Rights for the land, in her name alone, whereon she claimed: "The use of the waters of one Certain Creek, commonly Known as Deadman Creek, and by some known as Beaver Creek, to the extent of two (2) cubic feet per second." She needed this "for the purpose of Communicating power and the propagation of fish . . . and for irrigating . . . lands."

She accomplished this the month before James was killed, which was fortunate, because after his death, it was impossible *not* to question Mary's state of mind. It was the common opinion that she had not been "right" since James died. Given that Mary suffered a stroke following her son's death, which altered her mental capabilities, this is not surprising. Another result of the stroke was a decided limp, her body having also paid dearly following the shock of the traumatic experience. Some thought her brain was irreparably damaged. Despite this, Mary was summoned to court, ordered to produce James's last will and testament, and expected to behave as though she had all of her faculties. She longed only for her son.

Though Johnson insisted otherwise, Mary signed a sworn affidavit that she had no "knowledge or information that he ever made any will either in favor of the said Jennie H. Johnson or of any other persons." Mary stated that a different woman, Jennie *C.* Johnson, was the person who had lived with them and to whom James became attached. Mary related how shortly before James's death, he "suggested . . . that he would like to make a will and give the said Jennie C. Johnson a part at least of his property." Mary said she had acquired a book of legal forms and typed out different versions of a will to present to James, for his ultimate decision, but he died before this was accomplished.

—◆—

A witness was called from a law firm where Mary had taken the will. Under oath the man said that the paper she presented in court was not the same document he had previously viewed. The *Spokane Press* on August 16 described the seriousness of Mary's possibly self-inflicted predicament. The article leads with: "Punishment for contempt of court is awaiting Dr. Mary Latham if she persists in trifling with the orders of Judge Kennan to produce the real will of her son and all copies of it which she has made and all letters pertaining to it. The will in question, according to testimony given by persons who have examined it, gave all the son's $15,000 [more than $460,000 today] estate to his sweetheart, Jennie Johnson."

Inside the courtroom, stubborn Mary was making no friends. She swore, according to the *Press*, that "she had made a thorough search, finding the papers presented to the court today in a box upstairs over her store at Mead." Handwriting experts called to look at the will Mary presented claimed that "the ink on the document was not yet dry." Mary must have known that if she did indeed create a false will and was discovered, it would not go well for her.

The report continued: "She and the attorney got into a sparring match, Mrs. Latham refusing to answer. Mr. Latimer arose in his dignity and demanded a reply. 'Well, I don't know why I did it,' she said in rising voice and bringing her hand down on the counter with a thud. 'I don't remember anything these days.'" This statement may have come from a rare moment of clarity.

As the case proceeded, Mary's testimony took a bizarre turn. A witness swore that when Mary took the will to have it probated, she said, "Mrs. Johnson, the beneficiary under it, was a member of a royal family in Sweden, and that she neither cared for the property nor knew of its existence."

Based on the signed and sworn affidavits of two men, it was unexpected that Johnson had sued Mary for the estate. One man, W. H. Maloney, identified as an insurance agent. He had met Johnson in Mead while she was working at the Mead Mercantile Company, which he understood was owned by Mary. Maloney stated that "he wanted to make a survey of the store building and stock which he had already insured for Mrs. Latham; that it was then and there talked over and distinctly understood by the said Jennie Johnson, that the insurance was in the name of Mrs. Latham; that she made no suggestion or intimation of any kind that the insurance ought not to be in the name of Mrs. Latham as the owner of the property, but on the contrary spoke very freely of her business and interest there, and of her relation to the same and to Mrs. Latham; that she said she had no interest in the property."

Unfortunately, Maloney was identified on October 20, 1905, in the *Spokane Press* as being "under conviction in the federal court of illegal acts in connection with pension affidavits . . ."

The second man, Charles A. Prall from Mead, swore he was acquainted with both women. According to Prall, "he had a conversation with the said plaintiff in the month of June, 1904, in the course of which [Johnson] told [Prall] that she was intending to leave Mead soon . . . that she had no interest there and was not going to stay."

Johnson swore she had never had these conversations.

Prall had gone to Oregon for a time. He would become known as the man who captured four antelope for the Manito Park zoo "after many days of hard riding." When he returned from Oregon and was next in the company of John Messner, he was told of the lawsuit against Mary. He informed Messner of the conversation with Johnson, at which time the two men went directly to inform Mary's attorneys.

Charles Prall's marriage record lists his parents as John and Sarah Prall. John was likely J. W. Prall of Mead. It seems ironic that Charles would attempt to help Mary, while his father would employ the opposite tactic.

—◦—

Johnson claimed that Mary had written to her in Butte, Montana, asking her to come to Mead to live and work with her, and care for her in her final years. Johnson stated that Mary had promised to deed the property to her should she come.

Mary's attorneys filed an "Answer to Interrogatories" that she had been directed to provide under oath. In one she explained why Johnson came to Mead: "[Johnson] was homeless and not employed [and] I invited her to come to me with a view of helping her if she proved worthy and we got along well together." She also said, "I thought it might not advance my interest as a practicing physician to be conducting too many kinds of business in my own name and for temporary purposes only I took this title in her name." This perhaps shady practice of Mary's—though other records suggest it may have been a common one at that time—along with her habit of trusting the wrong people, led to her undoing.

Mary stuck to her story—that she "never wrote or stated to [Johnson] that all of the property James left was or would be hers." It was suggested in the interrogatories that Mary deeded the property to Johnson "for the purpose of defeating and defrauding your husband with whom you are not living, from taking as an heir of your son James A. Latham," though Mary had been divorced for nine years. Johnson asserted that Mary did this to defraud her creditors.

Mary vowed that Jennie Johnson had given her a power of attorney authorizing conveyance of the property at Mead. Indeed, a warranty deed was issued on March 25, 1904, conveying the land on section ten in Mead from Jennie H. Johnson to James G. Scribner. For Scribner's part, he swore "he never had any such deed in his possession, nor was there any notice given to him of such deed until he saw the same upon the records of said County, nor was same ever delivered to him, nor did he ever have knowledge thereof." The deed as recorded was transcribed as having been completed and signed as "Jennie H. Johnson, Per Mary A. Latham, Her attorney-in-fact." Perhaps Scribner was an innocent party.

Yet James G. Scribner was known to the Latham family. His name appears on deed records between 1902 and 1904; often purchasing land from James—until one month before James died—and subsequently selling it to Warren. There were also deeds between Scribner and Jennie Johnson.

Johnson filed an affidavit, per the *Spokane Chronicle* on August 23, "in which she alleges that she is the owner of the property in question; that she has no knowledge of the execution of any powers of attorney . . . never saw them, and that she can not successfully reply or defend the claims and affirmative defense without seeing said papers and making copies of them." Oddly, subsequent identical quitclaim deeds were filed on July 22 and August 2, at the request of the law firm of Barnes and Latimer, and by Jennie Johnson, respectively.

The preposterousness of Mary's testimony grew, perhaps due to a massive dose of anxiety. She seemed to be losing her grip on reality along with her hold on the property. Perhaps in a desperate ploy, the country of the Philippines entered her sworn statement. The *Chronicle* asserted: "Dr. Mary A. Latham states that she has practically won the will contest case . . . [and] that through the publicity given to the case by the newspapers she has found in the Philippines the Jennie C. Johnson, to whom she claims the property was bequeathed by her son, and is now sending to her the property intended for her." Mary must have understood how crazed her claim sounded to everyone in the courtroom. Though if she was suffering from what is today known as early-onset Alzheimer's disease, it's possible she did not.

The trial of Jennie Johnson against Mary Latham began on October 19, 1904. The Findings of Fact and Conclusions of Law signed by Judge Kennan on April 3, 1905, included the following: "That the plaintiff [Johnson] is entitled to a judgment for the delivery of the possession of said premises to her." On the same day, Attorney Kellam filed exceptions to each conclusion. Four days after the judge ruled in favor of Johnson, Mary's attorneys learned of the conversations that Maloney and Prall had with Johnson. As soon as the courthouse opened the next day, they filed an Amended Motion for New Trial, listing: "Newly discovered evidence material for defendants." Apparently it was too late. They were denied, and Johnson was granted ownership of the property.

Interestingly, fifteen days before Mary met Jennie Johnson in court, she deeded twenty-four city lots that she owned to her son, Warren, for a total consideration of one dollar. In 1911, she would deed four more city lots to Warren for the same price.

Following the devastating news that she would lose the land to Johnson, there would be no respite for Mary from her creditors. (Johnson would eventually file an $800—more than $24,000 today—damages suit against Mary for the burned building.)

The Spokane Drug Company joined the line of plaintiffs suing Mary in the spring of 1905, claiming that Mary "failed to pay for all of the drugs and supplies used in her profession." The statement reiterated that the company was suing "Dr. Latham for $83.26 . . . for articles purchased by Dr. Latham during the past two years and not paid for."

Once again, it could be supposed that this failure to take care of business was caused by Mary's ongoing grief and injured brain. What a mess she'd made. It was becoming apparent that she was a better caregiver than bookkeeper.

Open season had been declared on Dr. Mary Latham. Next sued for nonpayment of a book subscription by a publisher, she was then sued along with Edward for nonpayment of principal and interest by North American Loan & Trust. As a result of Mary's transactions—or lack thereof—with her creditors, coupled with the effects of her mental state, her credibility was waning. And her losses were accumulating.

CHAPTER 18

Fire in the Pharmacy

Fire at Mead early Sunday morning destroyed the building occupied by Dr. Mary Latham as a general merchandise and drug store. The stock, which was a small one, was almost entirely destroyed, little being saved. The origin of the fire is unknown. The building was owned by Miss Jennie Johnson, who secured the award a few days ago after a sensational suit.

The building had originally belonged to James A. Latham, son of the doctor, who, according to the evidence adduced, had willed it to Miss Johnson, to whom he had been engaged at the time of his death. When Miss Johnson appeared and claimed possession of the property, Dr. Latham contested the claim, setting up that the Jennie Johnson who claimed the property was not the same Jennie Johnson to whom her son had willed it.

The court awarded the property to Miss Johnson, but Dr. Latham continued to occupy it. It is rumored that Miss Johnson was to have taken possession today.
—Spokane Chronicle, May 8, 1905

Not one eyewitness came forward to say how or when the fire ignited in Mary's Mead Mercantile Company store.

A notable article appeared on May 9, 1905, two days after the fire. Spokane County sheriff Howard Doak had gone to Mead to investigate the fire. After returning to Spokane, Doak stated there would likely be no arrests made, and said, "While I was in Mead yesterday . . . I heard no suggestion other than that somebody set the place afire. There is no other cause known or thought of in the town."

Unfortunately for Mary, there would be an investigation, arrests, and a trial. The fire was only the beginning of the mess that would emerge from Mead to blacken Mary's reputation and utterly change her life as she knew it.

In a July 11 interview with the *Spokane Chronicle*, Mary claimed she had been threatened before the fire:

> *I didn't do it, that's all. We had some bitter enemies in Mead and just because we were getting along in business they threatened to turn us out and blow us up. A man came in the store . . . and, shaking his fist, said he would like to see the building burned and me in it. He also went on to say there was a scheme to send a minor in for liquor and get us into trouble that way.*

What about the intentions of the "bitter enemies" she mentioned? Was her story true?

Another tragedy would arise from the ashes in Mead. Above her business, Mary had stored safely away for posterity all of the adoption records for which she served as guardian. Finding homes of a high standard for homeless children had occupied much of Mary's life, and had brought joy to many childless couples in Spokane and the surrounding area. This was a truly staggering loss, though ten years would pass before the magnitude of the loss was truly understood.

On Christmas Day in 1915, two years before her death, Mary would be reminded of how fate can grab the reins and waylay the best, most carefully laid plans.

Mary was living on Spofford Avenue in Spokane when a thought-provoking case connected to her work with the Spokane Home-Finding Society became linked to the decade-old fire in the pharmacy.

In 1904 an infant girl had been brought to Mary for placement in a home. According to a newspaper headline—"Fortune Awaits for Little Girl"—this child was now a missing heiress. Regrettably, the only thing Mary could remember was that she had found her a home with "a farmer living somewhere near Spokane." Tragic for her many adoptees and probably embarrassing for Mary, the newspaper revealed that "all of the records of the society were destroyed by fire when a drug store operated by Dr. Latham at Mead burned."

One might wonder: If Mary *did* set fire to the building out of grief and rage, was there an additional compelling, misguided reason she might have done so? Was there something else that drove her, other than being ordered to relinquish the property to Johnson—perhaps the very fact that the Home-Finding Society child-placement records *were* stored there? However, all of these records must have borne the signature of the benevolent guardian, Dr. Mary Latham, attesting to the legal transaction.

In 1916, Mary would be instructed by a judge in relation to her home-finding service: "No action will be taken if she incorporates and conducts the business as [do] other similar societies." There is no indication what might have occurred to bring her before this judge.

The idea that Mary may have wanted to burn these adoption records carries little weight. As previously documented, Mary spent years caring for the children of Spokane, delivering babies and finding homes for the unwanted. She worked tirelessly for the little ones and their unfortunate mothers with compassion and devotion. It's more likely that in her 1905 state of mind, she forgot that the papers needed to be moved when she emptied the structure of her belongings prior to anyone taking it over.

CHAPTER 19

The Arson Trial

SPOKANE, Washington, June 23 [1905]—To the Editor [Spokane Chronicle]:

Your compassionate editorial under the head of "Dr. Latham's Jury," referring to the kind and humane recommendation of the jury, coupled with the sad and pathetic communication of Dr. Latham . . . recalls to [this] writer many scraps of her history in the past 15 years. . . . [S]he was left to struggle, single and alone, to support herself and family, and educate her three sons as best she could till they were able to look out for themselves. . . . Two were married and left the home roof, leaving the single one—James—who to her became her all. He was her chum—her adviser—her assistant—all that she had to lean upon.

One sad day he was rudely taken from her, losing his life by an accident in the railroad yards in this city. . . . Laboring under business duties and her profession, too onerous for a woman, and all the time overwhelmed with grief at the loss of her son, she came to labor under the impression—delusion, you may call it—that the whole world had turned against her. She has to her credit many genuine and unselfish acts of charity. Many of those she had sheltered and attended in their distress turned their backs on her, forgetting to even thank her. Is it not a wonder that her mind has not given away long ere this?

She is a woman in advanced years, and not a man, who has long battled with the asperities and mutations of fortune and steeled against the tide of misfortune.

With the network of circumstances woven against her, an honest jury could scarce have done otherwise than they did, but their hearts, with the pathetic figure before them, tempered their decision with a tender recommendation for mercy.

We all have our faults. She may have had hers. We are all human, and let us be charitable and drop a tear of sympathy for those whom circumstances of necessity have burdened, warped and embittered, their cherished hopes and ambitions destroyed and the results of a life's efforts ebbing away.

—PIONEER

There may have been others in addition to the mysterious "Pioneer" who felt sympathy toward Mary. Nevertheless, a warrant was filed in the Superior Court of Spokane County, on which Sheriff Howard Doak wrote: "I, H. B. Doak, Sheriff . . . do hereby certify that I have this 17th day of May 1905 arrested . . . Mary A. Latham."

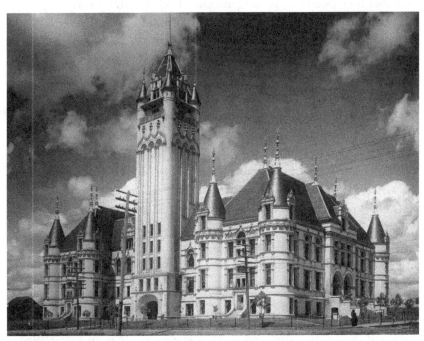

The stunning Spokane County Courthouse in 1905, suggestive of a French chateau.
NORTHWEST MUSEUM OF ARTS AND CULTURE / EASTERN WASHINGTON STATE HISTORICAL SOCIETY, CHARLES LIBBY COLLECTION, IMAGE L87-1.156

The June 10, 1905, edition of the *Spokesman-Review* stated the following: "Looking haggard and worn, Dr. Mary A. Latham yesterday began her ordeal in the superior court—the task of defending herself from the accusation of arson." This began a series of articles running for more than a week in the *Spokesman-Review* and other papers. Throughout the city—indeed, across the Inland Northwest—Mary's name was mentioned often, as it had been when she first arrived in Spokane Falls, although this time for scandalous reasons.

Mary was exhausted from all she'd experienced over the previous two years, and many who knew her believed her critical faculties had been deteriorating since the death of her son. No matter her state of mind, she was to be tried for arson, and would need to defend herself in Superior Court before Judge Miles Poindexter.

Leading her defense were attorneys D. W. Henley and A. G. Kellam. Together they faced prosecuting attorney Richard M. Barnhart.

Henley was eight years Mary's senior, and Kellam, seven. Would they bring the wisdom of age and experience to the courthouse in Mary's defense? The answer would come over the following days.

Henley had arrived in Spokane two months before the Great Fire of 1889, which destroyed his office building. Henley had "long been regarded as one of the leading lawyers in this part of the state." Kellam had "long been a careful and assiduous student of the law, and [possessed] a mastery of his profession to which few lawyers can hope to attain."

Henley and Kellam were connected outside the courtroom as well. An article published in January 1899 boasted: "Spokane is the mining metropolis of the northwest," further listing all mining companies incorporated in 1898. Henley and Kellam were listed as fellow incorporators of the Golden Lion Gold Mining Company, the Credo Mining & Smelting Company, and the Shenandoah Gold Mining Company.

As citizens assembled inside the courthouse for jury selection, Henley and Kellam quickly raised an objection. Richard Barnhart had presented the following proposition: "It may be necessary," he said, "for me to take the stand during this trial and make a statement. It is an extraordinary proceeding, but it may be unavoidable." It *was* extraordinary and generally allowed only under unusual circumstances. Against strong objections by Henley and Kellam, Judge Poindexter agreed to allow it.

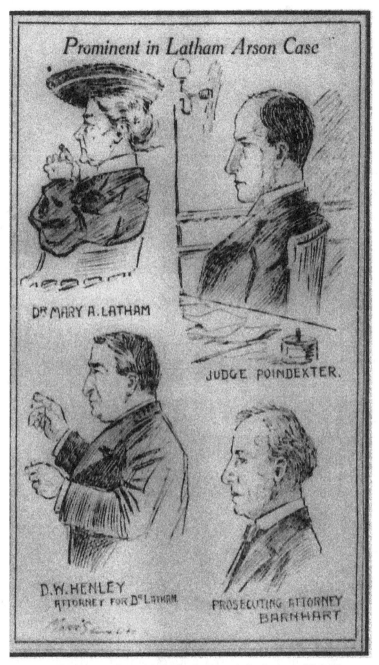

Prominent in Latham Arson Case

Dr Mary A. Latham

Judge Poindexter

D.W. Henley
Attorney for Dr Latham

Prosecuting Attorney
Barnhart

A pen-and-ink rendering, titled "Dr. Latham is in Serious Plight," depicts the prominent players in Mary's dramatic arson trial.

SPOKESMAN-REVIEW, JUNE 14, 1905

Following the second day of jury selection, a courtroom reporter noted that Mary would not look the selected jury members in the eye. Though she had maintained a strong professional standing in the community over the previous seventeen years, she may have felt like a stranger now, at the mercy of the all-male jury who would decide her fate. The jury members selected were: L. Baldwin, from Spokane; J. A. Baldwin, Spokane; J. J. Schaler, Medical Lake; A. P. Fassett, Spokane; Levi Allen, Spokane; H. D. Wright, Mount Hope; T. J. Jarvis, Latah; I. O. Worley, Spokane; J. S. Howard, Spokane; W. H. Blair, Rosalia; A. Patterson, Spokane; and John Steen, from Waverly. Aware that these dozen men would either restore her to her role as revered physician or remove her to the state penitentiary, Mary remained steadfast in her claim of innocence.

Hoping to turn Mary's fate in her favor, the defense team gathered a list of complimentary witnesses—or so they hoped. An "Abstract of Compensation to Witnesses" filed with the court listed the names of sixteen witnesses for the prosecution.

Immediately there was a problem with defense witness George Messner. George was the son of Mary's supposed accomplice, Dr. John H. Messner. John Messner had originally been accused along with Mary, but would escape prosecution for arson—although Mary would later stand against her traitorous friend.

George Messner was accused that he did "wilfully [sic], unlawfully, corruptly, wickedly and maliciously solicit, suborn, instigate and endeavor to persuade one Melvin [sometimes spelled Melville] Logan" to perjure himself in favor of Mary. Originally, Logan, who worked at Mary's livery, had been held inside the jail, also accused of "complicity in the burning of the store at Mead."

When a warrant was issued for George Messner, he did not appear. Attorney Henley "presented an affidavit signed by Dr. Latham that Messner was sick with gastritis and nervous prostration and could not appear in court." Messner previously told Mary and Attorney Henley that he overheard conversations between two witnesses for the prosecution, the details of which could shed light on the shadowy accusations against Mary.

A second affidavit was presented. This one signed by Dr. John L. Smith of Colbert, alleging the identical medical opinion regarding Messner, adding: "it would be extremely perilous to his life to attempt to bring him to Spokane."

Asking for a two-week continuance, Henley signed his affidavit, saying: "George Messner is a material witness for the defendant on the trial of this action . . . [and] he is the only witness so far as deponent [Henley] knows from which he can obtain information which it is necessary and essential for this deponent to have in order to properly cross-examine Nellie Stansbury and Melvin Logan." Mary had been told that Stansbury (sometimes spelled Stansbery or Standbury) and Logan would "testify to facts entirely different from and irreconcilably inconsistent with the statements made . . . to . . . [George] Messner."

Barnhart quickly called Deputy Sheriff J. M. Hone to the stand. Hone said he'd gone to Mead to find George Messner at home, where he lived on a lot adjoining Mary's. Hone saw Messner through a window, he reported, fully dressed in the sitting room with his wife. When he knocked on the door, Messner scurried up the stairs. His wife insisted Messner was "sick in bed and couldn't see anybody." Not to be deterred, Hone climbed the stairs, finding Messner under the bedcovers. He insisted the man get out of bed and come with him to Spokane.

Messner was furious, according to Hone: "Messner rose up in bed and got very angry . . . He said the officers were butting into the case too much. When I told him that I had been informed he had been up and around that day, he said that anybody who said so was a d——d liar." He refused to come without speaking to Mary first. Rather than argue with Messner further, Hone left him and returned empty-handed to Spokane.

Henley tried once again to influence the court to delay by stating other reasons Messner could not attend: His wife had just given birth; his oldest child had inadvertently been poisoned and nearly died; the strain of the aforementioned was too much for Messner.

The court was not convinced. "There is evidence here," said Judge Poindexter, "showing that this witness is able to come into court if he wants to. The motion for a continuance will be denied." Sheriff Howard Doak was sent to fetch Messner and brought him to Spokane to spend the night in jail, where Dr. George A. Gray examined him, declaring Messner well.

That day ended with these words: "There is a feeling around the courtroom that more sensations will be sprung before the case is over. In fact, the air of the courtroom is charged with electricity."

The crush of people in the courtroom may have gotten the jolt they were expecting when Mrs. Nellie Stansbury took the stand. One of Mary's employees at the time of the fire, Mrs. Stansbury was the first witness for the prosecution, earning a mention in the June 13 *Spokesman-Review* article headlined "Former Friend Hurts Dr. Latham."

Oddly, in a different newspaper accounting of when Sheriff Doak—with the assistance of Deputy Sheriff Pugh—went to arrest Mary and her employee, Stansbury was identified as "Mary Standbury . . . known later as Mrs. Scribner." This piece of information raises questions in relation to the previous Jennie H. Johnson trial, where it was learned that a deed had passed between Johnson and J. G. Scribner. Was this Scribner the future husband of Mary Standbury? Or was it Nellie Stansbury? Was this one woman, or two? Had a circle of friends in Mead conspired to get Mary's land?

Nellie Stansbury had been arrested under suspicion of aiding the accused arsonist, yet it wasn't long before authorities decided she was not involved, and she turned state's witness.

Reflecting the social environment of the time, the prevailing attitude toward women, as well as the standard for the pre–broadcast television era, one reporter wrote, "[Stansbury] is a slender, plain looking young woman, with raven black hair. While she does not appear overly intelligent, she demonstrated before the day was over that she could not be befuddled by the cross-examination of a shrewd attorney."

Asked to describe the store that burned on the early morning of May 7, Stansbury's description included Mary's residence—three blocks away from the fire—a livery stable owned by Mary, and a blacksmith forge nearby. Stansbury answered that her own home was on the Peone Prairie, where she usually lived with her mother and her brother, whose surname was Whipps.

Stansbury stated that she had known Mary for seven years, calculated from a time when her husband—who had been traveling between the Peone Prairie and Spokane—became ill and was taken to Mary for medical treatment. Stansbury later came to Mary's home to help care for him. Sometime after her husband recovered, Stansbury herself returned to Mary for treatment of an ailment. Practical Mary hired Stansbury to work in her home in order to pay for her treatment. She was still under Mary's employ at the time of the fire.

When questioned for a more detailed rundown of the store that burned, Stansbury explained that it had consisted of three businesses: a grocery store, a drugstore, and a general merchandise store. Next to the main structure stood a smaller building used as an office by Mary and shared with Dr. Messner, the veterinarian who was originally accused as her co-conspirator. There was a kitchen attached to the store, where Messner slept, and where Mary and her employees took their noon and evening meals. Gracious Mary provided breakfast for her employees inside her home.

When asked to recount what she remembered from that night, Stansbury testified to the following:

> *On the night of the fire I went to a dance at the brickyard about a mile from Mead. I went with Melvin Logan, an employee of Dr. Latham, and Emma Tibbetts, a girl of about 16 years of age. Melvin Logan drove us and we left the store about 8 o'clock. I stayed at the dance until after 12 o'clock. Melvin Logan and the Tibbetts girl left before I did. I came home with Charlie Harding. He had a horse, but I didn't know whether I could ride it or not, and we walked most of the way to Mead.*
>
> *When we got home it must have been nearly 2 o'clock. I went directly to the house and stood talking with Charlie Harding about two minutes, and then I went to bed. I noticed as we came by that there was a light burning in the store, which was unusual. There was also a light burning in the dining room of Dr. Latham's house, which also was unusual. I put it out before I went to bed.*

Stansbury continued, stating that not long after she'd gone to bed in Mary's home, there came a pounding on the door. According to the woman, when she opened it, there stood an agitated George Messner. "Come quick! The whole town's burning up!" Messner shouted. He quickly clarified his outburst, saying "The drug store's afire."

Stansbury swore that she went to Mary's bedroom and, discovering Mary wasn't there, proceeded to hurry outside. "I went on by myself. When I got there, I found Mrs. Latham standing by some pine trees and watching the fire."

"This is awful," was Mary's greeting to Stansbury, according to the latter's testimony. She swore that Mary was fully dressed and seemed to be alone.

Her further testimony revealed that Mary offered her gifts days after the fire. Stansbury described them as gloves, thread, and tobacco. She "told me to say I bought the stuff if anybody asked where I got it," Stansbury claimed.

———

Mary had never been afraid to speak her mind, although this time, it backfired. A witness named Mrs. Sadie Riley, described as "an exceedingly stout woman," proceeded to relate a conversation she'd had with Mary the previous autumn, when Mary had come to her home in Green Bluff to provide medical care.

A newspaper account quoted the exchange between Riley and the prosecutor:

Prosecutor Barnhart: "What conversation did you have with her?"
Riley: "Well, I asked her how her litigation with Jennie Johnson was coming on. She said she had won, but that Jennie had taken an appeal. I says [sic]: 'Well, she may beat you yet.' And she says: 'Well, if she does it won't do her any good: she'll never live in that store. She'll have to get up pretty early to beat Mrs. Latham.'"

Mary would come to regret her words with Riley—if indeed this was an accurate account—whether said out of sheer boastfulness or as a nod to something sinister.

——

After the fire, Mary apparently made odd requests of Stansbury, once asking her to fetch several rubber water bottles. Mary instructed her to fill them, place them on the floor to soil them, and then hang them in Mary's bathroom inside her home. Mary had given her no explanation.

Next, Stansbury claimed, Mary asked her to copy in her own hand a letter she had written to publish in the newspaper. This didn't seem far-fetched or unusual, Mary having published many essays and letters. What was unusual, Stansbury relayed, was what she saw when she reached the end of the letter: her own name. She refused to finish.

"It was a letter," Stansbury testified, "saying that the writer had known Mrs. Latham for 10 years; that she had always stood high in the communities where she had lived; that she was in bed the night of the fire, and that jealous enemies were trying to make trouble for her."

Coincidentally, an article appeared on May 10 with a statement purportedly given by Mrs. A. R. Smith of Mead, saying, "she knows that Dr. Latham was in bed at the time of the fire . . . [and that] Dr. Latham is the victim of jealous enemies." And yet, there was no Mrs. A. R. Smith called as a witness.

On the heels of Stansbury's testimony before Barnhart, Henley requested permission to interview George Messner, who was still in jail. He wanted to do this before cross-examining Stansbury, remembering that Messner had damning evidence about conversations between Stansbury and Logan. Henley insisted this was vital to Mary's case. Judge Poindexter refused the request. Without interviewing Messner, Henley tried but could not shake Stansbury off her testimony.

Henley proceeded to state that he would show how Mary had gained nothing by the destruction of the property. There was no insurance on the building. (It may be that the insurance mentioned by Maloney had expired.) Mary had a resulting loss of between $800 and $1,000 (more than $31,000 today). He would show that Mary was asleep at the time of the fire, Henley said, and that it was she who was awakened by the pounding of George Messner, not Stansbury. Furthermore, he declared that he would prove the defense witnesses "had been harassed and threatened with arrest by the prosecution, and that one of them had actually been arrested."

━ ‿ ━

Prosecution witness Clarence Binkley of Mead was next on the stand. Corroborating Stansbury's testimony, Binkley, a laborer also lodging in Mary's home (a common practice of farm laborers), swore that he did not see Mary when he woke and hurried out to the fire, testifying that he found the door unlocked and the house empty and that Mary was nowhere in sight. When he reached the fire, he said, he found her on the opposite side of the store from the house, fully dressed, watching the fire.

The prosecution made this conclusion: "To dress herself rapidly, and beat Binkley to the fire so badly that he did not even see her on the road—a three-block walk—and then to get around clear to the other side of the fire from her house before he arrived, was quick work, according to the theory of the [S]tate, for a woman as old and as slow in her movements as Dr. Latham."

━ ‿ ━

The evidence, though strictly circumstantial, continued to mount against Mary. On June 15, the newspaper reported that Dr. John Messner, her supposed friend, had not helped Mary's cause by confessing that he held a bill of sale for items Mary had already assigned to her creditors.

Once Messner finished his testimony, a notary named William D. Neidermeyer was called to the stand. Indeed, Neidermeyer swore that Mary had come to his office the previous month to make an assignment to cover debts to Spokane entities, such as "Holley, Mason, Marks & Co., the Ohio Wood company, the Crescent Manufacturing company, the Spokane Drug company, the Spokane Brewing and Malting company, James Durkin, and others."

━ ‿ ━

George Messner, still considered the star witness for the defense, was finally allowed to leave jail and come to the courtroom, where he endured stiff cross-examination by Barnhart, who chipped away at Messner's block of testimony.

Messner stated that he saw Mary standing in front of Cushing's ice-house at the time of the fire, fully clothed, even wearing her hat, watching the fire. Barnhart was quick to challenge Messner, reminding him that he had previously given a contradictory statement saying he had pounded his fist against Mary's door to sound the alarm, finding her wearing her nightdress with a skirt thrown over. How, Barnhart pressed, could she have so quickly been properly dressed at the scene of the fire if she had been sleeping just moments before? This was the question of the day. Another important question: Who was telling the truth?

It's possible that all the witnesses believed they were telling the truth—their truth. One person may recall the same event in an entirely different way from the next. Julian Matthews explains this phenomenon in his article, "Why Two People See the Same Thing But Have Different Memories," in *Neuroscience News*. The article begins: "Memory isn't perfect, and most memory differences are relatively trivial. But sometimes they can have serious consequences." Matthews continues, listing age, health, and stress as three contributors to poor memory retrieval. Memory perception is also influenced by a person's past experiences. "Retrieval is also affected by the outside world; even the wording of questions can change how we recall an event . . . [along with] the presence of other people. When groups of people work together they often experience collaborative inhibition—a deficit in overall memory performance. And of course, there are those 'tip-of-the-tongue' states—the common and frustrating experience that we hold something in long-term memory but we cannot retrieve it right now."

The next day's news was a bit salacious for 1905 Spokane. It concerned the widow Mrs. Annette Franzen and Dr. John H. Messner, with one sensational headline blaring "Messner Woos as Shop Burns." The prosecution insisted that Franzen explain her association with Messner. According to the article, "[Franzen] admitted that she allowed him to visit her frequently, knowing that he has a wife and family at Medford, Ore."

Franzen revealed the whereabouts of Messner on the night of the fire, telling the packed courtroom that he had arranged to spend the evening of the fire with her in her home.

Barnhart wanted more. He quizzed Franzen about Messner's marriage. She said it was a legal separation. He asked about Messner's family. She said, "He told me he was practically a free man."

Barnhart got to the point: "You and he are what we call in common parlance, lovers, aren't you?"

The defense objected, but Judge Poindexter directed Franzen to answer.

Franzen: "Well, he's been a friend of the family ever since we became acquainted."

Barnhart: "How long had your husband known him before he died?"

Franzen: "About three months."

Barnhart: "And Dr. Messner has been a friend of the family ever since your husband died?"

Franzen: "Yes, sir."

Barnhart: "And that family consists of you alone?"

Franzen: "Yes, sir."

<hr>

Henley called W. A. Glassen to the stand, hoping to impeach Melvin Logan, the star witness for the State. Besides stating that he had come upon Mary fully dressed and watching the fire, Logan had also testified that "two big cans of coal oil were brought to the store and placed in a woodshed at the rear of the store. The woodshed was burned, too."

Glassen stated that he'd heard Logan talking about the trial outside on a street in front of the Workingman's Home.

Barnhart cross-examined him: "Since Jim Hopkins disappeared out of this case you've been going about among these witnesses, haven't you?" The connection between Glassen and Hopkins is unclear. A local attorney who supported Mary and sat with her during the trial, Hopkins "was indicted by the federal grand jury at Seattle and left to attend to that urgent matter."

The case against Attorney James Hopkins would be settled later that year. Convicted of "making notorial acknowledgements without having the persons present in his office," a judge ruled no fraud had been committed. Hopkins was fined and forgiven, although his absence and the consequent lack of support during Mary's trial was another blow for her.

Barnhart plowed ahead with Glassen: "You're the man, aren't you, that Dr. Latham told down on the street corner the other day to be sure and have your boys swear to this thing?"

"Not in a thousand years!" Glassen exclaimed. "Anybody who says so simply lies."

—◦—

Finally, another laborer from Mead sat in the witness chair. O. H. Winkle testified that he had been asked by Dr. Messner to help move items from inside Mary's store, saying that he and Mary had "fallen out." (At least one account suggested Mary had feelings for Messner but was passed over for Franzen.) This transfer of items was done on the evening before the fire. Had Messner known something dreadful would soon transpire? His behavior might suggest so.

Winkle had been awakened by the fire, he said. It was *after* he reached the burning store that he saw Mary coming from her home. This was a positive point for the defense. Then, he added that she had been fully dressed, even wearing a hat. Unfortunately this was what Barnhart wanted to hear regarding whether Mary was fully dressed or not when alerted to the fire.

Once witness testimonies concluded, Henley made his closing statement. He clearly described having talked to Mary ten days before the fire about assigning her assets to creditors. On May 6, Mary visited Henley's office and signed the assignment, making one E. C. Gove the assignee. Henley then advised Mary that she and Dr. Messner should remove their personal items from the store before morning, when Gove was to take charge. With this information, it appeared Messner had simply been following Henley's advice. The following conclusion appeared in the evening paper:

The object of this latter testimony was to show why Dr. Latham and Dr. Messner removed their goods the night before the fire. The object in proving the assignment was to show that Dr. Latham had no motive in burning up the store, and that she was acting in good faith to pay off her creditors. The theory of the prosecution is, however, that Dr. Latham burned the store out of spite against Miss Jennie Johnson, who had beaten her in a lawsuit over title to it.

At 9:45 a.m. on June 17, 1905, Mary was sworn in for the fight of her life. Spokane's beautiful, pale brick courthouse was built in the design of a chateau, its tower looming high above the main entrance, flags waving from the central turret. Despite its castle-like architecture, it's likely Mary felt nothing like royalty. Seated in the dark, polished courtroom, she was examined and cross-examined until three o'clock in the afternoon.

Attorney Henley approached Mary first, asking preliminary questions. To these she answered that she had been a practicing physician for twenty years; that in 1904 she had moved to Mead to live and work; and that before this time she had lived and practiced her profession in Spokane.

"How long have you known Dr. J. H. Messner?" Henley asked.

"About a year."

"How did you become acquainted with him?"

"I was called to treat him professionally. His ankle was crushed," she replied.

Mary attested that Messner had moved his drugs and himself to Mead as soon as he was well, setting up his business. At first this may have seemed like an advantageous arrangement: having a veterinarian on hand to care for her valuable mode of transportation, her horses.

Mary agreed with the statement that Messner had removed his possessions from the store as advised by Henley, as had she, and that this happened on the night before the fire. She also agreed with witnesses whose statements declared they had seen lights burning late into the night in the store.

I left a light turned down in the back end of the store," Mary said, "secured the doors and went home. George Messner, who lives just north of me, overtook me on the way and walked home with me. The distance was about two blocks and a half."

"What did you do when you reached home?" Henley asked.

"I went to bed."

"Had Nellie Stansbury returned from the dance?"

"No, sir."

"Did you leave a light burning?"

"I did."

Mary explained that she had not undressed when she went to bed. She affirmed she had only removed her overskirt and her "high elastic slippers," that she was in bed about two minutes after reaching home, and that she was awake when Stansbury came in. She continued by saying she heard George Messner coming to arouse her and that she had subsequently called out to Clarence Binkley. Mary stated that she immediately returned to her bedroom, put on her skirt and elastic shoes, and went to the fire. She elaborated:

> When I first got to the fire, I stood by the barn and watched it until it got too hot there. Then I went farther east by some pine trees, and stood there and watched it. When I got to the fire Melvin Logan, George Messner and O. H. Winkle were there. Mrs. Stansbury arrived 15 or 20 minutes after I did, and from then until the fire burned down she and I were together. We went home together after the building was consumed. I don't know just what time the fire occurred, but it was getting to be daylight when it was over. The building was consumed in half an hour.

To close his questioning of Mary, Henley was succinct: "Did you set it afire?"

"I did not."

Next, Mary endured Prosecutor Barnhart's examination. He brought to light every possible detail to make Mary look suspicious, careless, and scheming. He prodded her to admit how her insurance policy had expired and no longer covered the store. That the insurance company did not consider the store a good risk because of the previous litigation against Mary by her creditors. She agreed that the insurance coverage had expired, admitting she had since tried to be extra careful of fire.

Barnhart's suspicious questions followed:

"But you had a fire in the stove that night before the building was burned, didn't you?"

"Yes, sir."

"And you went away and left it burning?"

"The stove was still hot; there was little fire there."

Barnhart accused Mary of not being concerned about what she had lost in the fire, of not seeking to retrieve coins that had melted in the blaze, and of not seeking out and informing the sheriff. He also accused her of creating the creditors' assignment as a convenience prepared in advance of the fire.

He questioned her once more about the heart of the issue. "Dr. Latham, do you know anything about the origin of the fire that burned up that store building?"

"I have not the slightest idea how it started."

Mary was next questioned about a bill of sale she had given Dr. Messner. She explained that she had paid him $100 (more than $3,000 today) each month to watch over the store when he could.

Barnhart was skeptical. "And you got his services for $100 a month only for such time as he could be in the store?"

"That wasn't all," she replied. "He looked after the ranch for me."

"What ranch?"

"My son's ranch."

"What would he do?"

"Well, he would direct work to be done on it."

"Couldn't you do that?"

"No."

"You were paying out of your own money for the care of your son's ranch?"

"Well, my son and I are one," said Mary.

"Oh!" was all Prosecutor Barnhart could manage, and the courtroom was dismissed for lunch.

Reporters must have scurried to their offices to file their stories. Some newspapers were rife with sarcasm regarding Mary's testimony. Others were more understanding of the long-idolized physician.

⁓

Modern clinical studies reveal what might have saved Mary in another time. One scientific publication states: "Our review suggests that individuals with PTSD, a history of trauma, or depression are at risk for producing false memories when they are exposed to information that is related to their knowledge base. Memory aberrations are notable characteristics of posttraumatic stress disorder (PTSD) and depression." The article explains that there are several ways "to evoke suggestion-induced false memories." Perhaps a persistent, antagonistic prosecutor was too much for Mary's traumatized brain.

⁓

Steadfast in the belief of her innocence, Mary must have grown wearier with each passing day. One might imagine her fear increasing daily as one witness after another testified against her. Not so, apparently; she believed in the process and in her innocence, later saying that she had not been afraid because she carried no guilt. She listened while her life was laid bare to a room full of neighbors and friends who had held her in high esteem over the course of two decades. She'd been a pillar of the community. She'd saved countless lives. Would those truths count for nothing inside the courtroom? Would anyone save Mary?

Clearly, it would not be the prosecutor, if he was successful.

Barnhart pushed Mary to finally admit to writing the letter she had tried to get Stansbury to sign and deliver to the newspaper office. Then, he turned to the subject of Jennie Johnson, a painful one for Mary.

The testimony below contains the first reference identifying Scribner as "Dr." Either Barnhart was unaware he used the term, was getting confused between the names Messner and Scribner, or perhaps this was an error of the press.

Barnhart: "You deeded that property to Jennie Johnson, didn't you?"

Mary: "I had it deeded to her by the man from whom I bought it. I put it in her name on condition that she would stay there and live with me."

Barnhart: "Afterward you deeded the property to Dr. Scribner?"

Mary: "Yes."

Barnhart: "How did you do that?"

Mary: "I had Miss Johnson's power of attorney. She was trying to rob me."

Barnhart: "Was there any consideration [payment] for the deed to Dr. Scribner?"

Mary: "No."

Barnhart: "Did Miss Johnson know you were deeding it to him?"

Mary: "She did not."

Barnhart: "And you mean to say that you used that power of attorney to deed Miss Johnson's property away without consideration?"

Mary: "I did it because it was really mine, and she was trying to rob me."

It was becoming more obvious by the day that Mary's view of the world in which she lived was skewed, perhaps presenting like a hall of mirrors in her mind, with her wondering which direction to take in order to avoid crashing into herself, shattering her view of the world? Would the jury recommend mercy? Would Judge Poindexter grant it?

Repeatedly, Mary faced the presentation of circumstantial evidence, each witness giving a slightly altered version of what happened, a bit like the old game of "Telephone." She was again interrogated about the stove in the store, what she wore to bed, who awakened her, who was present when she approached the fire. Barnhart asked why Mary had not awakened the Cushing family, whom he said lived close enough to be threatened by the fire. (W. G. Cushing's name appears on the "Abstract of Compensation to Witnesses" form in the case file from Mary's trial, indicating he was summoned to court.)

"My thought was that Dr. Messner was asleep in the burning store, and I wanted to find out about him," Mary said.

"If he had been asleep there he would have burned to a cinder by that time, wouldn't he?"

"I don't know."

"As a matter of fact," Barnhart continued, "after you arrived at the fire you didn't mention Dr. Messner's name to a living soul, did you, or inquire about him?"

"I think I did."

"Whom did you inquire of?"

"I don't know."

Facing the aging physician, Barnhart announced that he had no more questions.

⤙⤚

Mary was showing her age, and it was no surprise, especially with the added stress of the trial. In spite of her frailty in her coming final decade, and all that would occur during this terrible week and beyond, she would outlive Prosecutor Barnhart by seven years. Barnhart was killed in a railroad accident near Everett, Washington, on March 2, 1910, when the train he was riding in tumbled two hundred feet to the bottom of a canyon, pushed by an "ice slide." Buried under thirty feet of snow and ice, he was one of eighty-four people who died. Mary outlived Henley's partner, Kellam, by four years, when he died of kidney disease. Henley survived Mary by four years.

Only Judge Miles Poindexter survived well beyond the trial, living to become a congressman serving eastern Washington. Senator Poindexter later announced he was running for president of the United States. At least one person doubted Poindexter. Interviewed by the *Chronicle*, former president William Howard Taft, while waiting to board a train for Spokane, was asked if he thought Poindexter would succeed in earning the Republican nomination for president. "You are not asking me seriously, are you?" was Taft's response. When the reporter replied that he was, Taft said, "Well, then I'll have to answer you seriously . . . If Poindexter's candidacy has any strength, I have failed to discover it." Apparently, Taft was right.

In the evening following the wind-up of trial arguments, the final paragraphs of a lengthy news article described how things stood:

> *The theory of the [S]tate throughout the trial was that Dr. Latham burned the store out of spite over Miss Johnson's victory in the courts. Dr. Latham's defense was an alibi, mainly. She also tried to prove that she had no motive for burning the store, and that when the fire occurred, she was perfecting an appeal to the supreme court.*
>
> *Dr. Latham is a pioneer physician of Spokane. She is about 60 years of age and has two grown sons and one dead son. She is divorced. Her husband is a government physician in the Indian service, and lives at Nespelim, [sic] Washington. She is partly paralyzed, and walks with a pronounced limp.*

Closing arguments had concluded, the clock was ticking, and everyone in the courtroom—likely in the entire city—anxiously awaited the verdict.

Henley and Kellam tried to postpone what now seemed inevitable by filing a motion for a new trial, stating: "First: Error of law occurring at the trial and excepted to by the defendant; Second: That the verdict is contrary to the law and to the evidence."

Would the woman who for seventeen years had been a saint for sick women, unfortunate girls, and homeless children and infants be condemned to prison? Would the one who had tended the minds as well as the bodies of Spokanites be put on a train to Walla Walla and the state penitentiary? Conviction for the crime of arson could bring a sentence of up to ten years in the penitentiary. What would Judge Poindexter rule if Mary was pronounced guilty?

Surely a hush fell over the packed courtroom on June 18, 1905, as the jury shuffled in, so that everyone could hear the verdict. It had taken twelve men a little over two hours of deliberation to arrive at one decision: guilty of arson. The verdict statement was handed over with a handwritten plea across its face: "With recommendation to the leniency of the Court" signed by L. Baldwin, her fellow trustee of the Union Library Association.

Reportedly Mary remained stoic in the face of the devastating pronouncement. But neither she nor anyone else would hear her sentencing that day; that would have to wait.

Mary left the courthouse in the company of her son, Warren.

While Mary awaited sentencing, Governor Mead raised a question about management at the penitentiary in Walla Walla: Should a matron be appointed for the sole care of the women's department? Did this idea relate in any way to the fact that the esteemed Dr. Mary Latham was likely headed there?

Later that year, in November, the governor's "board of control" appointed Mrs. Ella Goodman to the new position. She would receive a salary of $50 (more than $1,500 today) per month.

Mary was not inert while awaiting sentencing. She returned to her familiar form of expression: a letter to the editor. On June 22, 1905, the *Chronicle* published it under the headline: "Says Her Dead Son Comes Back Each Night."

In part, Mary wrote:

Being in feeble health and knowing that death may come at any time, I wish to make the following statement, which, as I hope for forgiveness, is true. This is in reference to the fire . . . Melvin Logan told several people who can be readily produced that I was not at the store that evening of the fire. Afterwards he said he told the story [in court] that he did in order to save himself.

I've been called insane by a score of people and I've wandered [sic] if I am. Since the tragic death of my son two years ago, he has never failed to come to me nightly, sometimes as a little boy, sometimes as a six foot man, and I may be insane, but there is a comfort in this that they can not take away.

While awaiting the summons for her sentencing appearance, Mary rested at the home of friends, the Posey family. One evening, she abruptly announced that she was going on the streetcar. Mrs. Posey described what happened: "The doctor got away from me and went down to the Sprague avenue car and went down town [*sic*]. I telephoned the police and they brought her back. She was not trying to get away, simply went downtown with the idea of throwing herself in front of a train and meeting her death in the same manner as her son, James, did."

Mary had recently expressed suicidal thoughts. Now, muttering and crying and causing a scene, Mary rode the streetcar to the corner of Riverside Avenue and Howard Street. Officer Miles of the Spokane Police Department was waiting for her. Miles boarded the car with the intention of removing Mary to bring her safely home, but she wanted no part of that plan. She was convinced James was awaiting her arrival either downtown or somewhere out in the great beyond. She fussed and wailed and protested until Miles carefully but firmly escorted her off the streetcar. Weeping, Mary was taken to the police station. When she finally quieted from exhaustion, confused by the actions of others, she was sent safely home an hour before midnight in a horse-drawn hack. The ordeal left her friends and the police officers believing "her mind has been shattered by the ordeal through which she has passed."

Later, she would tell an interviewer while convalescing at the Posey home:

I've been pretty sick and I wish I could get well. . . . I keep thinking my boy will come back. He comes sometimes—only for that I wouldn't want to live at all. I went to town one night to find him—his train came in at 10:45. They wouldn't let me go. I don't think that he is dead at all.

I don't have anything to do but lie here and think and think. I know a good deal about drugs and have thought out a restoring fluid which, if applied at once, even when one is seriously injured, will keep them from dying. Here is a letter I have written to the undertaker asking him if Jim is there. I saw him there last, and if he had had some of this fluid he could have saved Jim—but I do not believe it was Jim at all—it was some one else.

What else would one need to attest to the state of Mary's mind?

On June 19, Henley and Kellam had filed a statement by Dr. D. C. Newman regarding Mary's overall health. Newman verified that "said defendant is in a very nervous condition and is suffering with a severe pain in her head and is threatened with a second stroke of paralysis; that she has heretofore suffered from one stroke of paralysis; . . . [and] that it would be perilous to the life and health of said defendant to . . . attempt to bring her into the presence of the Court."

It's interesting to note that on June 23, five days after hearing her guilty verdict and soon after her attorneys filed Dr. Newman's statement regarding the precarious state of her health, Mary deeded 520 acres in Mead to W. A. Glassen—one of the witnesses for the defense—for $6,000. The price of about $12 per acre for land already developed was quite a bargain for Glassen, with raw agricultural land selling for over $20 per acre.

On the day of her sentencing Mary was expected in court, no excuses allowed. The *Spokane Press*, on July 20, gave a detailed account of the outrageous manner in which her sentencing played out: "Lying on a stretcher on the floor of the criminal department of the superior court, Dr. Mary A. Latham was sentenced by Judge Poindexter." Four deputy sheriffs had each gripped a corner of the stretcher bearing Mary and carried her inside. At the direction of Poindexter, she'd been brought by ambulance from the Posey home to the front door of the courthouse. Mary was said to be "lying in a state of apparent semistupor [*sic*]." Few citizens would witness this, for the court had purposely kept quiet when she would appear.

Mary later explained to an interviewer how she came to be in such a state:

The shock which I sustained upon hearing the verdict of the jury was so great that it absolutely prostrated me, and I have been in a very miserable condition ever since. The shock was all the greater from the fact that neither myself, my attorney, or my friends had the slightest idea that there would be any result of the trial other than my unconditional acquittal. . . . There being no guilt, there was consequently no fear, you see.

I am in receipt, daily, of letters from all over this section of the country from old friends and patients, expressing their sympathy and belief in my innocence. Letters have come from British Columbia, Seattle, Tacoma, Portland, and from ever so many smaller towns, the gist of them all being that the writers could not and would not believe me guilty and tendering me their heartfelt sympathy and hoping that the final outcome of the case, even though it looks so dark at the present time, will be in my favor.

Attorney Henley approached Judge Poindexter to announce that he intended to file a new motion in the case. Poindexter asked if anyone had anything to say regarding whether the sentence should not be pronounced. It was reported Henley stooped over Mary where she lay on the stretcher, and she quietly replied, "Nothing but that I am not guilty."

Judge Poindexter said, according to the *Chronicle*, that Mary's trial "was one of the most aggravating that had ever come under his observation, calling attention to the defiant attitude of the defendant during the trial." Was she actually defiant, or merely sticking to the truth of her convictions?

The only other moment Mary spoke during her sentencing hearing was to say, "I came here looking for my boy. Is he here?"

Henley was convinced the court was in error for refusing to admit certain testimony. He also claimed he was not given enough time for summarizing a case lasting seven days, and where circumstantial evidence was the only kind submitted.

Mary had not been well when the trial commenced and was feeling worse now. Henley recognized this and tried to convince the court to send her home to recuperate rather than to prison. He believed that "to sentence her at this time would be a serious menace to her life." He believed she had earned that consideration. "I have known the defendant for the 16 years I have been a resident of Spokane," Henley said, "and I say here that no more gracious acts have been committed by any 25 women in Spokane county. No day has been so disagreeable, no night so dark, no patient so poor that this defendant was kept from the bedside. She is a woman of the largest feelings for humanity."

The *Chronicle* detailed Henley's plea for Mary:

Other errors alleged were that the court had failed to give an instruction on motive, although he had been requested to do so by the defense, and that he [Poindexter] had unreasonably limited the attorney's [sic] for the defense to two hours which to argue the evidence before the jury and said that this act on the part of the court had been an abuse of discretion and had worked a hardship upon the defense.

Attorney Henley also laid great stress upon his claim that the evidence was not sufficient to justify the verdict, and in arguing this point asserted that at least two of the [S]tate's witnesses had been compelled to testify as they did in order to save themselves from prosecution for the very offense of which Mary was convicted. He argued that the evidence was entirely circumstantial, and that if ever a conviction was secured in a court of justice through malice, prejudice, hatred and perjured testimony, this was the one. He closed his argument by declaring that if the case could be retried by a jury of citizens of Spokane, the result would be different and the defendant would be acquitted.

Poindexter was not moved. "In this case there is absolutely nothing to recommend leniency," said the judge, "except the consideration of old age. The sentence of the court is confinement in the state penitentiary at hard labor for a period of four years, and to pay a fine of $1,000 [more than $31,000 today] and the costs of prosecution."

Mary was going to prison. If she stirred from where she lay on the stretcher, it was not recorded. Perhaps she was in a state of shock. Returned by ambulance to the Posey home, some were skeptical when they saw Mary on a stretcher. Only she knew whether her collapse was a genuine result of the trauma of the past two years or a guise—one last attempt at finding mercy.

——⁓——

It was the end of August in Spokane when suddenly a grand jury was called and Mary was brought before them. Shockingly, she confessed that as a culmination of everything that she'd experienced over the two years since the death of her son, James, she had, along with John H. Messner, set fire to her store at Mead. She explained that she and Messner had punctured a coal oil can repeatedly, used it as a sprinkling can, and "saturated the premises with coal oil."

"Mrs. Latham has had an unending amount of trouble over her property," reported the *Spokane Press*, "and she claims further that she thought the store was hers and that she had a right to burn it and that she did it because she believed she was being greatly wronged by persons whom she thought were trying to rob her of her property." The paper added, "It is believed Warren Latham, Mrs. Latham's son, used his influence to persuade his mother to make the confession."

Was this because Warren believed—or knew—that she was guilty; or did he influence her to say she was guilty, mistakenly believing it would end the ordeal and she would receive probation? The latter seems unlikely when considering Warren's upright life of service. In the end, after the prolonged trial during which Mary had several times declared her innocence, often displaying reticence, she admitted to the madness of which she was accused.

——⁓——

But then, what of her suspected co-conspirator, Dr. John H. Messner? If he was innocent, why was he suddenly gone from not only Spokane County, but from the state? The *Lewiston* [Idaho] *Inter-State News* on August 4 announced that Messner was "Wanted on Arson Charge." The article stated: "Deputy Sheriff Charles Monroe arrested Dr. John H. Messner last evening and is now holding him at the county jail awaiting the arrival of an officer from Spokane, where Dr. Messner is wanted to answer the charge of arson in connection with the Dr. Mary Latham case."

Seven days later the newspaper updated readers as to the situation surrounding Messner, saying, "The habeas corpus [writ presented to a judge to secure prisoner release] was dismissed and the judge remanded the prisoner to the custody of the sheriff to await the arrival of the extradition papers."

Why did Messner, after acting suspiciously, ultimately escape prosecution for the charge of arson, while a woman who had tirelessly dedicated herself to her community and its citizens for nearly two decades—who had experienced extreme life-altering trauma, was possibly suffering from early signs of dementia, and most certainly suffered from depression—should receive the sole and severe punishment?

CHAPTER 20

Fugitive from Justice

Spokane Press, July 28, 1905:

A story was started and received some credence to the effect that in the initial stages of her flight the doctor had left a farewell message to a physician friend.

This story originated in an alleged telegram which had gained some circulation among people who have been discussing the case. A Press reporter has seen a copy of the telegram. . . .

The alleged telegram is probably the result of the lucubrations [meditation] of some joker. The message reads as follows:

The good doctors who had me dying and taken into court on a stretcher are entitled to my heartfelt thanks, and so, while on the wing to escape officials, I stop long enough to send this message: My professional brethren and friends, when I think of the noble and unselfish action of the good brother who made me a two-time paralytic and then fed me on "strawberries only" for weeks, I feel that I can never repay the kindness of the profession. If I am caught I shall expect you and others of our great profession to make any statements necessary to shield me. Inform our friends that I am feeling well.

—DR. LATHAM

Someone had it out for Mary. Evidently, there were some who thought Mary's behavior a ruse. In truth, the "telegram" was the ruse.

First, how likely is it that someone considered a desperate fugitive would stop long enough mid-flight to write a telegram of any length? And would they stop to remove the addressee from the telegraph form after sending it—and why? The regulation form examined by the *Press* reporter had the addressee section cut away from it. The whole idea seems a bit absurd. Secondly, the message was signed "Dr. Latham." It should be mentioned that in various essays and more than thirty letters to editors, Mary signed her name to include either her initials, her first name, or a combination thereof, once using her initials only, "M. A. L.," for a postscript. She never signed as "Dr. Latham." That, after all, was her once and only husband's moniker.

Facing incarceration, Mary fell under the persuasion of two men and supposed friends, John W. Prall and the disreputable Dr. John Messner. Succumbing to their coaxing, Mary made what was feasibly the worst decision of her life. The men assured her that if she would only provide them with a certain sum of money, they would access records and buy off the prosecuting attorney and the judge, sparing her a prison term. They convinced her, according to Barbara F. Cochran in *Seven Frontier Women and the Founding of Spokane Falls*, she need only leave town for five years, at which time she could return to practice medicine, safe from prosecution.

Surely horrified by the thought of enduring a prison term—or dying there—Mary followed the ill-fated instructions of the two men, escaping in the bottom of a wagon, according to reports. Arriving at her home in Mead, she reportedly spent the night there before heading alone toward Idaho. The same paper later clarified that no one saw her in Mead, after all. Either way, staying just ahead of tailing law enforcement, Mary may not have been traveling solo. Accompanying her, according to one account, were her supposed friends, Dr. John H. Messner and Mrs. Annette Franzen. One witness reported that Messner had stated he would be leaving Mead, possibly for two weeks, possibly never to return.

Reportedly, once the group reached Rathdrum, Idaho, Messner and Franzen cruelly disappeared. The abandoned Mary must have been bewildered. Yet, solitary in her purpose to adhere to the plot devised by Prall and Messner, she continued on alone.

"Where is Dr. Mary Latham?" began an article in the *Spokane Press* on July 25, 1905. "A wild rumor came swinging across the northern end of the city and struck the courthouse today that the erstwhile sick, bedridden physician and convicted arsonist had skipped the country."

On August 1, the *Press* published a succinct account of Mary's desperate race for freedom. Common conjecture was that she was traveling cross-country to the Mississippi River, where she would sail down the river and find her way to Mexico. If this were true, would she not have headed south and east? Instead, once her "friends" Messner and Franzen had deserted Mary, she'd taken her horse by the reins and turned the buggy north. She drove until she found herself surrounded by a forest of lodgepole and ponderosa pine, western red cedar, spruce, and Douglas fir. It might have been a lovely setting for a lonely woman, if only she weren't lost.

In her mind, Mary was setting out on a camping adventure. More than once over the years, local newspaper tidbits had announced that Mary was away camping with one or another friend or family member. She would later say that this time she'd gone to meet old friends from Cincinnati. However, no one was seen in her company, save her dog. "A camping outfit," her valise, a fur wrap, and spare shoes had been stowed in the buggy.

Eventually, she would reach a part of northern Idaho where "the home of an elderly gentleman named Schroeder was chanced upon." Apparently, Schroeder answered Mary's inquiries as to where to find a good camping spot, but the grade to get there was too steep for her horse and buggy. She drove on until she found a different route on Sheep's Hill. According to the *Press*, she entered "a part of the wildest and densest forest imaginable . . . [where she] drove between trees so close together that both were barked [*sic*] by the passing hubs of the wheels."

It was when Mary rested on her third night in the forest that her sorrel horse escaped. Breaking away from the buggy and dragging its tether, in two days' time the horse had found its way back to Rathdrum, where it "fell into the hands of Sheriff Doust, furnishing him a clew to the whereabouts of the doctor." The reporter does not reveal what the *clew* was.

Mary's mind may have been exhausted with trying to sort out her thoughts. Perhaps one minute she was convinced she was looking for a camping spot, and the next minute, she was certain she must flee. Either way, the determined Mary was not about to let the absence of her horse stop her. It was reported that she eventually lost her lovable mutt to the forest as well. The sixty-year-old woman set out on foot the next day, and in the end she traversed the forests of northern Idaho alone for a total of seven days and nights.

Mary took to visiting ranches in the area, looking for water, sustenance, and shelter. Though the ranches were far removed from Spokane, and the area sparsely populated, when Mary walked onto the ranch owned by Schroeder, he knew who she was. Word was surreptitiously sent to the sheriff at Rathdrum. But Mary didn't stay.

Next, she discovered the Jim Moseley (sometimes spelled Mosely) ranch in the Hoodoo Valley. She'd been searching for her horse, needed a place to rest for the night, and by now, needed another horse. She and Moseley were working out a price for a fresh horse when—thanks to Schroeder's message to the sheriff—two deputies arrived. "When captured Dr. Latham was eating dinner at the cabin of a bachelor named Mosely," reported a Walla Walla paper. Having been sent from Rathdrum after the Schroeder sighting to search for Mary, the two deputies had stopped to ask for lodging. Imagine their surprise when they walked in and came face-to-face with the "dangerous" fugitive.

The two Kootenai County deputies, Merritt and McDonald, asked Mary to return to Rathdrum with them, which, their report pronounced, she " 'was only too glad to do,' expressing surprise that a search had been made for her for a week." The three went to try to recover her buggy. No easy search, her buggy was found a reported three-quarters of a mile off the main road. Searching through scrub and downed trees, Mary's extra pair of shoes and her valise were also located. She said she'd hidden them 20 yards away (it was actually closer to 150 yards, according to the deputies). The article concluded: "This is considered to be pretty good proof that the woman had become confused."

While Mary waited in Rathdrum for the sheriff from Spokane and the southbound train they would board, she was interviewed by a *Tribune* reporter. Although she insisted she had not been trying to escape, it begs the question: Why had she climbed into the bottom of a wagon to get out of the city unseen, if that report were true? Mary asserted that she "had a good bond [with the court] and had no idea that it would prevent her from coming over into Idaho for two weeks' camping." She insisted that her Cincinnati friends had been with her.

Had she hallucinated the experience, or was this a convenient fabrication of the "facts"?

Mary was probably thinking about her original bond with the court, but the *Chronicle* reported that "the bond was not renewed at the time sentence was imposed . . . At the time the bond was first required it was signed by Warren Latham, her son, and Mrs. Louise Kellogg."

The interviewer for the *Tribune* continued, stating that the Spokane doctor had expressed "a boundless admiration for that growing city." He wrote that Mary "is not unprepossessing in appearance and has a kindly expression . . . She appeared fatigued but cheerful."

Spokane County sheriff Howard B. Doak had started for Rathdrum as soon as he learned Mary had been found—the second time Doak was on his way to arrest Mary.

Reportedly, when Mary saw Doak, she said, "That's a familiar face . . . and I guess we'll go right on home now."

There followed a simple statement: "Monday . . . night Sheriff Doak and Dr. Latham were passengers on No. 3, bound for Spokane."

It's fortunate that Mary did not run or resist when deputies first appeared. Members of law enforcement had been instructed to bring Dr. Mary A. Latham back—dead or alive. This proclamation seems outrageous, declaring that deadly force could be used against a befuddled, unarmed, sixty-year-old woman who had never hurt another person.

The court held a different opinion of Mary, thanks to the influence of Messner and Prall: a prisoner in danger of fleeing again. On August 2, a motion was filed with the court by Prosecuting Attorney Barnhart asking for "an order increasing the bond on appeal . . . to the sum of Ten Thousand Dollars [more than $300,000 today]." The motion described how the defendant "was allowed to go at large" and "had fled from the justice of the State of Washington." To support his request for the exorbitant

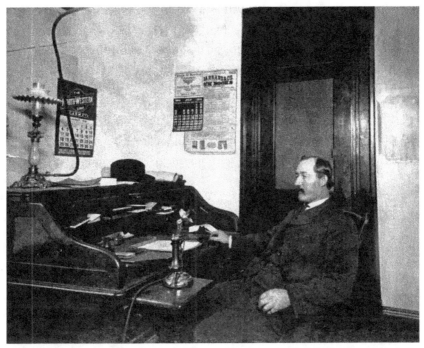

The Spokane County sheriff who first arrested Mary, Howard B. Doak, at his desk.
COURTESY OF THE ERIK HIGHBERG COLLECTION

bond amount, Barnhart explained how law enforcement had "pursued a vigorous search for said defendant, and after a continuous search, running over nearly two weeks of time and the expenditure of considerable money . . . said defendant was . . . arrested in the mountains of northern Idaho." Mary's time on the run was one week and a day.

Once Mary was back in Spokane and confined in the county jail, she described how the duplicitous "J. W. Prall and J. H. Messner had made overtures to her that if she would turn over to them a certain real estate mortgage for $3,650 [more than $113,000 today], they would arrange with the court, so she would not again be apprehended."

The two men were arrested, tried, and convicted of conspiracy to defraud. In October 1905, the *Spokane Press* closed a lengthy article regarding their trial with this: "The jurors betray signs of having occupied the jury box for a long time. Not a man there but what presents the appearance of having entered into the first stages of raising a full beard. A magnificent crop of mattress material is in the making."

Prall and Messner were fined and sentenced to jail—Messner for six months, and Prall for one year. However, neither man would be required to serve out his sentence. Messner received a commutation from Governor Mead, and Prall appealed to the Supreme Court. The court freed him, since the sole witness was Mary, with no one to corroborate.

CHAPTER 21

Prison Blues

SPOKANE, Washington, February 26 [1907]—To the Editor of the Chronicle:

Having recently received (unsolicited by me) a "full and unconditional" pardon for an act I never committed, and having been, according to a statement made by a prominent court official, "acquitted by the whole community months and months ago," I now ask for space in your paper in which to set to rights a few misstatements which have been published in several papers repeatedly....

All of this trouble came after the sad taking off of my son ... which left me ... a "mental and physical wreck." I went about as one in a dream ... living alone in our home on Fourth avenue. Inside the house were the pictures he had hung, the rugs he had laid. In the yard were the trees he had planted, the grass that grew from the seed his hands had sown, and I could not turn without expecting to see him....

[A]nd I here take the opportunity to offer $500 [more than $14,000 today] to any one who can produce any tangible uncontrovertible [sic] evidence that I did do so. Further, I wish to say that I offer to any one who will cause the arrest and conviction of the parties who did it the sum of $1,000.

Never in my whole life have I willfully wronged a fellow being, and as my friends all know I am always ready and willing to assist any one in trouble (often to my detriment).

But it is worth all I have gone through to know that beyond question the best people of Spokane county are my best friends and that they show their faith daily by financial, social and moral support, and the

fact that I am assured that the whole community "acquitted me months ago," is a very comforting one.
    —*DR. MARY A. LATHAM*

In November of 1905, Mary was still in the Spokane County jail. The *Spokane Press* explained, "Dr. Latham is serving time here in Spokane which will count on her penitentiary sentence, because she is retained here to avoid transportation expenses from Walla Walla when desired as a witness in forthcoming trials."

After the first of the year, though, the news Mary had probably been dreading was delivered to her cell: She was being removed from jail to the penitentiary.

On the morning of her departure, the newspaper read, "Aged Physician Leaves the County Jail in Company with Thieves, Hold-Up Men and Other Dangerous Criminals." The reporter seemed compassionate, describing Mary thusly: "The most pathetic figure of the eight who were taken from the Mallon avenue entrance to the county jail to begin the journey to the sinister walls of the state penitentiary was Dr. Mary A.

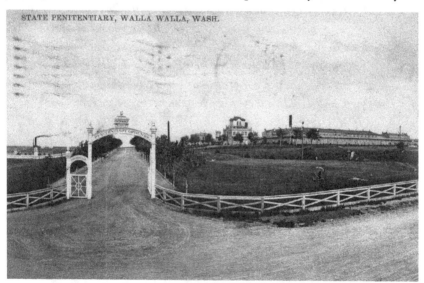

STATE PENITENTIARY, WALLA WALLA, WASH.

A postcard image of the prison gate in Walla Walla through which Mary passed in 1906.
COURTESY OF THE BEVERLY HODGINS COLLECTION

Latham, convicted arsonist, and at one time one of the foremost citizens of Spokane." He described her as "an aged woman" who "ate sparingly." Reportedly, she delayed getting dressed until assistance was sent to make her ready to join the line of convicts awaiting a shuttle to the railway station. Mary had left an impression. "Even the officers," he wrote, "had a kind of sentimental tenderness for the aged physician." Ever polite, it was reported she "managed to choke out a 'good-bye' as she was leaving."

On January 9, 1906, in frail health, Mary walked unevenly through the doors of the Washington State Penitentiary in Walla Walla. Undoubtedly, at that moment, Mary felt very far removed from the farmer's daughter she'd been born—tromping through the fertile fields of southwestern Ohio as a girl. Housed within the brick walls of the Women's Quarters behind locked doors, she was inmate number 4009.

Mary's mug shot is proof that even upon entering prison, she cared about her appearance. Her hair, though a bit disheveled, is atop her head in a bun. She wears earrings and what appears to be a mink or fur collar or coat. Her convict's personal property form completed at the time of

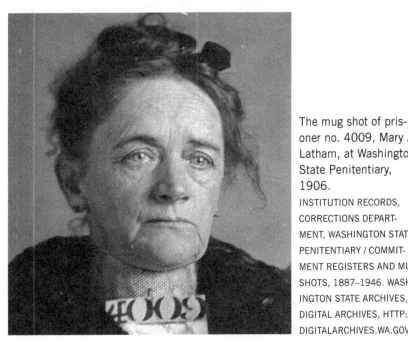

The mug shot of prisoner no. 4009, Mary A. Latham, at Washington State Penitentiary, 1906.
INSTITUTION RECORDS, CORRECTIONS DEPARTMENT, WASHINGTON STATE PENITENTIARY / COMMITMENT REGISTERS AND MUG SHOTS, 1887–1946. WASHINGTON STATE ARCHIVES, DIGITAL ARCHIVES, HTTP://DIGITALARCHIVES.WA.GOV

processing lists, "one pair gold glasses, one piece pink lace, one piece blue lace, one of thread lace, one of white silk finish, one handmade Batenburg [*sic*] handkerchief, and papers." Below the words *Signature of Convict*, the form was signed "Mary A. Latham," and below *Signature of Officer*, "Mrs. E. Goodman." This was the same Mrs. Goodman appointed as the first matron of the penitentiary during Mary's conviction year. Oddly, the form is dated December 21, 1906, when records show Mary arrived in January. The date of January 9, 1906, is written on the description of convict form, which was completed next.

Had Mary objected when prison officials measured parts of her body? They described her as 5 feet, 6 inches tall with light brown hair (described as dark brown on her mug-shot entry), with blue eyes. The form recorded the diameter of her head—7.2 inches; the distance between her temples—5.8 inches; the length of her nose—2 inches; her chest—41 inches; her forearm—10 inches; "elbow to point of middle finger"—19 inches; "width of hand at knuckle joints"—3 inches; "length of middle finger"—4.8 inches; and the length of her foot—9.4 inches. Her teeth were described in this way: "All lower teeth that remain, gold browned, upper teeth all gone, use[s] false ones."

American law enforcement had adopted this identification system, called "The Bertillon System," after its creator, French police officer, Alphonse Bertillon. The system was "based on physical measurements, individual scars, marks and tattoos, and personality characteristics." This is in part why Mary was subjected to such strict scrutiny, being imprisoned at the end of a period during the late 1800s and early 1900s, when "science attributed criminal behavior to physical defects and measured body parts to support that theory." Mary's mug shot remarks under "Marks and Scars" were as follows: "Mole on right temple. Mole on left side of chin. Mole on left cheek bone. Left 5th finger enlarged at 2nd joint."

Mary's carriage was described as "erect." Even on her worst day, Mary kept her bearing. Upon reading the form, it's obvious there was something amiss. Mary reported she was fifty-four years old, but having been born in November of 1844, her actual age at the time was sixty-one. Then, she gave an address for her nearest relative, her son Frank—who was living in Spokane—as Richland, Ohio. Perhaps she was confusing the name of Richland (a city in Washington) with New Richmond (Ohio), where Frank was born.

There may have been no obvious physical defects other than her noticeable limp, but her health, already fragile, was said to worsen during her incarceration. Consequently, with less than two years served of her four-year sentence, she was granted parole by Governor Mead in March 1907, to become effective April 1.

Two months before her release, an article had been printed in a Walla Walla newspaper revealing important information regarding Mary's temporary home. The following facts appeared: "Discussing the moral and physical welfare of the convicts, present and future, at the state penitentiary at Walla Walla, the report of the committee of investigation appointed by Gov. Mead read as follows: 'In brief, we do not consider the moral and physical conditions of the convicts at present satisfactory, nor do we believe it possible to appreciably better their conditions . . . until by legislative enactment.'" The committee reported this statistic: "Sex of convicts on hand—Males, 828, females 12." One of the twelve was Mary.

Could there have been a reason Mary was released early other than her poor health, or the results of the above-mentioned investigation? Mary's attorneys, Henley and Kellam, worked tirelessly to persuade Governor Mead to bestow executive clemency on Mary. The two men, along with fellow Spokanite supporters, were convinced that Judge Poindexter had not treated her fairly during her sentencing, under the persuasion of a long-held grudge.

Apparently, in 1901, when Poindexter was a deputy prosecuting attorney, he failed to win a verdict of manslaughter against a woman named Bertha Wardrum (also spelled Woodrum), charged with murder by abortion. According to Mary's attorneys, this failure of Poindexter's was attributed to the testimony of the chief witness for the defense at that time: Dr. Mary Latham. In court records from the Wardrum trial, Mary's name is among several witnesses, including other doctors, who were subpoenaed to appear at the Superior Court on May 7, 1901. However, while testimonies of a few of the doctors were transcribed into the court record, Mary's was not found.

Poindexter was not happy having failed to convict Wardrum, a midwife practicing in Spokane. On several birth certificates signed variously as "Bertha Wardrum," "Mrs. B. Wardrum," and "Mrs. Bertha Wardrum," she neglected to strike through the initials "M.D." printed on the form and write in the word "Midwife" instead, which was the practice of the day. Wardrum had also been accused of "holding herself out to [the victim] as a physician and surgeon."

Poindexter had begun the year 1901 more than unhappy with proceedings in court. In January 1901, the *Spokane Chronicle*, under the headline "Free Fight in Court: Attorneys Poindexter and Frank Graves Mix Up," reported: "Poindexter during this time was not idle. He was making a grand effort . . . when the crowd closed around. In a last effort he made a reach for his opponent, but whether the blow landed or hit someone else there is no record on the court docket to show."

There was more.

Besides Mary having a presiding judge whose opinions, the attorneys believed, were adversely influenced by Mary's connection to this past event, someone had been allowed to serve on her jury who should not have been.

Henley and Kellam reported what happened when one of the jurors from Mary's trial was approached for his signature on a petition for clemency. He "declared he would not [sign], that she ought to have got a life term and that he always had been prejudiced against her and was surprised that he had been put on the jury." In a later report, the man denied this statement.

Yet, even after being circumstantially convicted of arson, detained in both the city and the county jail, and taken to the Washington State Penitentiary to serve out her sentence of hard labor, Mary still had friends and admirers. Evidence of this appeared months before parole was granted, with a plea for pardon posted in a notice of support in the *Spokane Chronicle*, on July 18, 1906. It began, "An appeal to the women of Spokane to assist in obtaining mercy from Governor A. E. Mead for Dr. Mary A. Latham."

Life began to improve for Mary once Governor Mead granted her early parole. A statement summarized the decision: "[It] is represented by the prosecuting attorney, [S]heriff [Doak] and citizens of Spokane that the woman has been sufficiently punished and her release is recommended. The prisoner is 60 years old, with health and mind failing, and her son agrees to furnish her a comfortable home."

Mary returned to her beloved Spokane, having been paroled on April 1, 1907. She dutifully completed her parole report forms every month while staying with son, Frank, and his wife, Emma, in their home on College Place. During the months of April and May, when reporting she had worked for Frank doing housework, Mary signed her name under the printed closing salutation "Very Respectfully." Below this was a line for the signature of her employer; this is where Frank signed. Crossing out the word "Employer," he substituted the words, "First Friend." A US Department of Justice parole commission report explains: "U.S. Marshals were used as parole supervisors when needed. A system of monthly reports by parolees and the 'first friends' was initiated."

On May 22, Mary wrote to Warden M. F. Kincaid about her desire to work:

Dear Sir,
I write to ask if it be in any way out of place for me to have an office [in Spokane] for the practice of my profession (medicine)? My old friends and many new ones are anxious for me to do so. My home of course would be still with my son and everything be in keeping with the conditions of my parole, but I could then be able to earn quite a sum of money. Which I very much need as my pretended friends, lawyers et al. have robbed me unmercifully. Will you kindly let me know as to my privileges in the premises [appears to mean near her son, Frank's home]? My son and his wife are very kind, and my health is very good.
Very Respectfully,
Mary A. Latham
P.S. My son is willing for me to open an office, which will probably [be] in connection with the drug store in which he has an interest. M.A.L.

Warden Kincaid replied positively to Mary's request, placing Mary's letter on the desk of his secretary with a note of instruction attached: "Tell her she may do so with pleasure." This type of reply would not have been sent to someone who was seen only as a disrespected felon.

Once Kincaid granted Mary permission to return to her profession, her parole report forms listed her employment as "the practice of medicine."

⁓

Soon after returning to Spokane, Mary—strong in spite of everything—made a revealing statement:

> I never was in better health in my life, though they paroled me because they said I was in failing health and failing mentality. I don't look very crazy, do I? I have had a fine rest and do not consider the penitentiary sentence as a disgrace. It was only an instance. I shall hold my head just as high as ever.

⁓

Nearly a year later, a news item with a touch of sarcasm was published:

> Mary A. Latham, sentenced to four years for arson, is another applicant for executive clemency, as is J. H. Messner, now serving out the $500 fine that was part of the sentence given him in October last year for conspiring to defraud Mrs. Latham. It is a peculiar fact that in the Latham petitions it is charged that Messner and his partner [Prall] improperly influenced Mrs. Latham to commit the crime she is paying the penalty for, while the Messner application pictures Messner as an innocent, kindhearted old man, who wouldn't do a thing wrong.

The State Board of Pardons met in January 1908 to consider giving final discharge, pardon, paroles, and commutations of sentence to a group of convicts. Under the title, "Final Discharge," the *Evening Statesman* reported: "The following eight prisoners who are on parole have been

recommended for final discharge for the reason of their exemplary conduct while on parole: . . . Mary A. Latham."

Exemplary conduct . . . Mary excelled even when it came to being an
inmate. She was to be exonerated, and must have experienced a great
sense of relief.

CHAPTER 22

At It Again

The song [was] sung . . . in a voice filled with pathetic tenderness—the voice of one whose life had been one of burdensome cares, and weary heartaches—yet [it was sung as if by one] who felt a hope . . .

The feeble wail of a newly born child was the next sound to greet my ears—so feeble indeed that no one save the young mother and myself had heard it. The wail of a bit of humanity so small and ill-formed that I was glad to notice that the cry became feebler, and the breath grew shorter—then the wailing and the breathing stopped.

Poor little one.

The sick young woman was left for a time to rest, the tiny body of the dead baby removed, and not one person in all of that great lodging house, where people were passing to and fro at all hours of the day and night, knew that there had been a soul added to their number or that it had departed so soon after.

—MARY A. LATHAM, "The Story of a Song," Spokane Review, September 20, 1891

Many years had passed since Mary experienced the incident described above. She had endured much, persevering when others may have faltered. Now, only one year after her parole had been granted, a headline blared from the front page of the *Spokesman-Review* in 1908: "DR. MARY LATHAM AGAIN BEHIND BARS: Noted Woman Ex-Convict Faces Criminal Practice [Abortion] Charge." A harsh lead-in to the article, but true nevertheless: Mary was once again in custody at the county jail.

Had she become extraordinarily careless? Was dementia completely taking over her mind? Did she think herself above the law, or was she simply vulnerable to persons she felt were in need of her care?

One of her patients, a Mrs. Harrison, had caused a warrant to be issued against her. Pressing the charge of "criminal practice," Harrison declared that she had been taken to Deaconess Hospital in the spring, ill with blood poisoning. Blood poisoning, she said, "as a result of an operation performed on her by Dr. Latham." Harrison claimed that of necessity another physician had been called to perform a life-saving operation on her.

Mary told her side of the story: "The young woman came to me for treatment early in the spring and I gave her a room at my home, keeping her there for several weeks. One day when I went home she was not there, and I found she had called a cab and gone to the rooming house on Monroe street, near Boone avenue." She added, "Mrs. Harrison left my house a well woman May 4, owing me about $100 [more than $3,000 today]."

The *Spokesman-Review* reporter described how Mary was dressed when she exited the jail cell to provide this statement. "Dr. Latham was neatly, even jauntily, attired in a summery suit of white, with insertions and things and a flowery hat, which she wore, even in jail." Mary posted bond of $1,500 (more than $44,000 today), and the charge against her was dismissed. One can imagine Mary walking from the majestic courthouse in her "summery suit of white," head held high.

As has been established, Mary—ever sympathetic to women's causes, particularly health care for women and girls—had a soft spot for young women who were unmarried and pregnant. The words *pregnant* and *abortion* did not generally appear in newsprint during the years Mary lived in Spokane. Unwed pregnant girls were usually described as "unfortunate" or "betrayed," as having come to the big city to "hide their shame." Even in one of Mary's dispatches from Alaska, describing a future hospital's purpose, she reported the planned hospital would, in particular, stand ready to accept what the locals called "shipwrecked girls."

The social mores of the day did not condone abortion, although it was sometimes necessary to save the life of a mother after a botched attempt. Physicians often found themselves in the news and sometimes in the courts after attempting to save one of these women.

Mary had spoken out about this issue in the past. In an article published in September 1903 in the *Chronicle,* the word *abortion* is never used. Under the headline, "Give the Doctors Justice," it states:

> *In a communication from Dr. Mary A. Latham, she states with reference to current gossip as to criminal operations, that in a great majority of cases the women have brought themselves into a condition where the physician is compelled, whether he wishes or not, to complete the work already commenced. "It goes without saying, that no physician solicits business of this kind, and all abominate it, but all are unwillingly, and sometimes unwittingly, drawn perforce into it, and then they must and will of necessity do the very best that can be done with the case, for humanity's sake."*

In 1910 Mary was once again accused, suspected of performing an abortion. As usual, the word was not used; instead, the act was identified as a "criminal operation." The article in the *Spokane Press* in April 1910 began, "More sin and sorrow are brought out in new development in the Rose Elliott police scandal." The article described the woe that had come upon "the unfortunate girl for her weakness, her pregnancy [finally this word is used] and the removal thereof . . .

"From an affidavit made by Mrs. Dr. Mary A. Latham . . . Rosie Elliott turned up there between the 25th of February and the 1st of March and said that she was pregnant and had been so for three or four months. Dr. Latham made an examination and confirmed the girl's report and gave her some medicine."

Mary explained that the medicine she gave was to combat nausea, and for nothing else, which, of course, is taken to mean something that would have induced miscarriage.

Because of Mary's work with the Spokane Home-Finding Society and because of the advanced term of the girl's pregnancy, it seems reasonable to believe Mary's testimony in her affidavit. The reporter for the *Press* gives a lengthy description of the girl's activities, suggesting that she "was relieved of her trouble in some way between March 1 and 31, when she entered the hospital. Who performed the operation? Who paid the medical attendance?" He added that there were "people now trying to cover up the facts in the Rosie Elliott case."

The reporter gave an account of a visit he made to a Miss Van Duzen, who ran a home for expectant women. Van Duzen insisted she knew nothing of the case, or of how Rosie Elliott was "relieved of her trouble." She threatened to have the reporter arrested. About Van Duzen it was said, "She was very indignant and grew extremely wrathy when questioned as to her knowledge of the case."

Unbelievably, but perhaps by now to be expected, Mary was charged with abortion again the following year. From the files of the court:

Said defendant, Mary Latham, on or about the 18th day of November, 1910, in the County of Spokane and State of Washington, then and there being, did then and there unlawfully, feloniously, and wilfully [sic] use a certain metallic instrument upon the person of one Florence Stauffer, said Florence Stauffer then and there being a pregnant woman, with intent then and there to commit and produce a miscarriage of said Florence Stauffer, the same not being necessary to preserve the life of said Florence Stauffer or that of the child whereof she was then and there pregnant.

Though there were half a dozen witnesses against Mary, the case was dismissed in March 1911. The Motion and Statement explained:

Comes now the prosecuting attorney and moves to dismiss this case upon the grounds and for the reason that in the opinion of the prosecuting attorney, in view of all the evidence in the case, there is a strong probability that a conviction might not be had, and for the further reason that the defendant in this case is an aged woman and in broken health, and desires and is willing to retire from active life, and the prosecuting attorney is informed by a reputable physician that the defendant's mental condition is very much impaired.

CHAPTER 23

The Final Years

SPOKANE, April 5 [1911]—To the Editor of the Chronicle:
    Referring to the Stauffer case, of which the public has heard frequently of late. I would like to say that when the poor little girl came to me last fall she was unable to stand up for long at a time, and when she told me her pitiful story, the same old one of girls' trust and men's perfidy, I advised her to marry the man who had wronged her. She replied that she could not, as he was already married, and, besides that, had left the state.

    She then told me . . . [drugs] had been furnished her by persons who had been a party to her downfall . . . I then wrote down her statement just as she had made it, asked her to read it. She did so and I asked her if it were true. On her reply that it was I asked her to sign it, which she did without hesitation.

    I did this . . . as a means of self-protection, blackmailers, like the poor, being with us always.

    I have given up my offices, and, owing to failing health, will give up general practice. I will also give up all charity work except the home-finding work, it being one of my greatest pleasures to secure homes for the homeless little ones.

    No one need ever come to me with a hard-luck story from now on, as the story will be met with a deaf ear.
    Respectfully,
    —DR. M. A. LATHAM

It was 1911 and Mary was ready to relinquish her many passion projects, except, she was clear, the home-finding work. And, as the year was coming to a close, Mary was planning to travel again.

"Dr. Mary A. Latham announced . . . she intends to leave Spokane for the [C]anal [Z]one about January 1," stated the *Spokane Chronicle* in November, "and will be there for some time." Perhaps Mary was in accord with Mrs. Mary A. Garbutt, who was interviewed for the *Tacoma Times*. In an article titled "Women Want Panama to be a Monument of Peace," Garbutt expressed concerns sparked by government plans to send US troops to protect the Canal Zone. She had high hopes to move "the women of the West to try to induce [C]ongress to leave the Panama [C]anal unfortified and to erect at its entrance, in the place of cannon and forts, a gigantic statue of peace." Garbutt believed that "to fortify the canal is to invite attack."

No evidence was found that Mary fulfilled her desire to travel to Panama. She was likely too frail.

Mary may not have traveled to Panama, but plenty of guests traveled to stay with her in her Spofford Avenue home in the year 1912. Between September and December alone, the papers reported five women from "Idaho, Montana, and Lewisville [*sic*], Kentucky"; a couple from Idaho; a professor who came from his home state of Missouri; and "Captain and Mrs. C. W. Child . . . [who announced] the arrival of a baby daughter, born at the home of Dr. Mary Latham."

In the fall of that year, Mary purchased land that would remain with the Latham family for over a hundred years. The *Spokesman-Review* shared the good news: "For $10,000 [more than $280,000 today] Dr. Mary Latham has purchased through the office of S. A. Smart, Rookery building, 160 acres of farmland at Long Lake. The property at present is chiefly unimproved, but it is the intention of the buyer to make considerable improvements. Among other things, she expects to erect a sanitorium on the property and will also set out an extensive orchard." Mary's land was located less than two miles from Long Lake, which divides an adjoining section of land as it snakes for two miles through the terrain.

Near the end of 1916, just months before her death, Mary was summoned to court. This time it had nothing to do with land, but rather with her home-finding association. Judge Blake questioned her concerning the Society, for which she was still seeking infants for adoption. A November article in the *Semi-Weekly Spokesman-Review* reported that she had appeared in juvenile court, but that "no further steps have been taken in connection with her activities. It is expected no action will be taken if she incorporates and conducts the business as other similar societies."

As 1917 dawned, Mary, still gracious as ever, opened her home on Spofford Avenue to Mr. and Mrs. Charles Augustine, likely to assist Mrs. Augustine while giving birth. Sadly, the tiny infant soon became ill with pneumonia. Mary, of course, offered to attend the baby. Despite Mary's sensitive care, wee Velma Elizabeth Augustine died. Soon after, Mary contracted the disease herself. While waging a valiant battle against the infection, and despite the care of a colleague, the disease overcame her tired body and her weakening will. She was finally taken to Sacred Heart Hospital.

In the very place she had brought about healing for others, with her grandson, Hesper, and his mother, Emma, at her bedside, Dr. Mary Archard Latham died on January 20, 1917.

"Dr. Mary A. Latham Dead; Came to Spokane in 1888" read the headline in that evening's issue of the *Spokane Chronicle*. The following obituary stated: "Mrs. Latham was connected with various benevolent societies of Spokane and was one of the prime movers in establishing Spokane's first public library. . . . [She] was head of the Spokane Children's Home [and] conducted a woman's hospital in Lidgerwood . . ."

An article posted on the Fairmount Memorial Association website observes, "The final years of Mary's life were undeserving for such a kind and caring woman."

Inside the pages of the *Directory of Deceased American Physicians, 1804–1929*, Mary's "type of practice" is listed as "Allopath," which is a physician who uses conventional means (i.e., drugs) to treat disease. However, in December of 1889, Mary had posted an advertisement that read: "For pure homeopathic medicines go to Dr. Latham's dispensary." Some of Mary's life—including her medical practice—remains a mystery.

⌐⌐

Less than a month after her death, the *Spokane Chronicle* announced that pioneer Mary had died intestate. Leaving no will with instructions on how to dispose of her estate—valued at $3,000 (more than $63,000 today)—this left son Warren responsible for seeking letters of administration from the court in order to distribute the estate to him and his older brother, Frank, her immediate heirs.

⌐⌐

Respectfully described by Bragg in *More Than Petticoats*, at the end of her life Mary was "remembered as a pioneer woman physician of great civic involvement . . . all else seems to have been forgotten."

⌐⌐

When Mary's ex-husband Edward died in Chelan, Washington, in 1928, the headline read, "Friend of Indians Dies." In spite of the lifelong achievements and recognition both doctors achieved, the headstone at the Latham gravesite reads simply: *Edward H. Latham, and Mary, his wife*, along with each one's year of death. Neither of them remarried, and in the end, they lay side by side once again.

⌐⌐

A bronze bust of Mary's likeness was installed in 2003 as one of twelve "Builders and Leaders," significant contributors—three of whom were women—to the development of early Spokane. Located in downtown Spokane, they are the work of sculptor Wayne Chabre, from Walla Walla, and were commissioned by the *Spokesman-Review*.

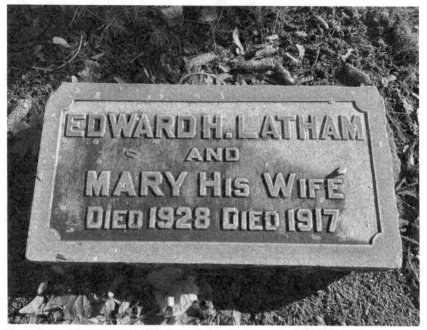

The headstone of Edward and Mary Latham at Greenwood Memorial Terrace in Spokane, Washington.
COURTESY OF THE BEVERLY HODGINS COLLECTION

On April 4, 2007, a larger monument to Mary—more befitting than the simple headstone—was donated by the Spokane Police Department History Book Committee, the Spokane Law Enforcement Museum, and the Fairmount Memorial Association, and placed near the three Latham family members interred at the Greenwood Memorial Terrace.

In the *Spokesman-Review* of November 13, 2019, Mary's name appears in print in the article, "Best and Brightest: Spokane-Area Women, Past and Present, Blaze Trails." A description of Mary's life of service, along with those of several other women, is part of a section entitled "Early Influencers."

These testaments to the astounding work and remarkable life of Dr. Mary Archard Latham prove that her legacy, even if tarnished, endures to this day.

BIBLIOGRAPHY

Sources used only in passing are not included in this bibliography.

"1900 United States Federal Census—Ancestry.com—James A. Latham." search.ancestry.com/collections/7602/records/73251940.

"Abandoned Baby Dies: Dr. Mary Latham Tells of Girl's Betrayal." *Semi-Weekly Spokesman-Review.* July 24, 1910. newspapers.com/image/566207586.

"After 16 Months, Mrs. Nancy Lemmerhart [Lammerhart] Released from the Medical Lake Asylum." *Semi-Weekly Spokesman-Review.* May 25, 1895. newspapers.com/image/566361741.

"Aged Woman Is Paroled: Mary A. L[a]tham is Given Her Liberty from Penitentiary." *Evening Statesman* (Walla Walla, WA). February 28, 1907. newspapers.com/image/194805088.

"American Humane: First to Serve." americanhumane.org/about-us/history.

American Medical Directory: A Register of Legally Qualified Physicians of the United States, 3rd ed. Chicago: American Medical Association, 1912. books.google.com/books.

"Appointed Physician at Colville." *Seattle Post-Intelligencer.* December 16, 1890. newspapers.com/image/332705835.

"Appointment." *Chicago Tribune.* January 20, 1875. newspapers.com/image/349263922.

Archerd, William F. *Archerd: Family History*, 2nd ed. lulu.com, 2015.

"Are Ready to Quit the County Farm." *Spokane Chronicle.* March 13, 1908. newspapers.com/image/561734486.

Armitage, Sue. *Shaping the Public Good: Women Making History in the Pacific Northwest.* Corvallis: Oregon State University Press, 2015.

"Arrest Made in Arson Case: Melville Logan Held for Complicity in Latham Fire at Mead." *Semi-Weekly Spokesman-Review.* May 12, 1905. newspapers.com/image/566290921.

"Arts—Photographs." *Lebanon Express*. March 24, 1981. newspapers
.com/image/414980150.

"Ask Her Release: It Is Claimed that an Inmate at Medical Lake Is Not
Insane." *Semi-Weekly Spokesman-Review*. April 28, 1895. newspapers
.com/image/566357421.

Atchison Daily Globe (Atchison, KS). April 22, 1893. 4.

"Baby Show: It Will Be Made an Attractive Feature of the Fruit
Fair." *Spokane Chronicle*. September 11, 1897. newspapers.com/
image/562117649.

"Baby Show for the Fair: Prizes for the Prettiest Infants in the
Town." *Spokane Chronicle*. October 6, 1899. newspapers.com/
image/561487842.

"Baby Will Probably Die: An Accident which Occurred on Monroe
Street This Morning." *Spokane Chronicle*. (1891c, March 21). news-
papers.com/image/562159777.

"Back from Dawson: Spokane Woman Who Braved the Terrors of
Chilkoot." *Semi-Weekly Spokesman-Review*. October 16, 1898. news-
papers.com/image/566367031.

"Ball Opened: Drs. Reddy and Carey Arrested for Practicing Medicine
Without a License." *Spokane Review*. July 18, 1891. newspapers
.com/image/565836280.

Bamonte, Suzanne, and Tony Bamonte. *Life Behind the Badge: The Spokane Police Department's Founding Years, 1881–1903*. Spokane, WA:
Tornado Creek Publications, 2008.

"Best and Brightest: Spokane-Area Women, Past and Present, Blaze
Trails." *Spokesman-Review*. November 13, 2019.

"Better Go Out of Business: Committee Recommends Orphans' Home
to Give Up Its Work." *Spokane Chronicle*. April 5, 1909. newspapers
.com/image/562078006.

"Biochemic College." *Spokane Chronicle*. September 26, 1891. newspa-
pers.com/image/562931303.

"Board of Education: Reports—Appointments—Resignations—Great
Lack of Room for Pupils—Condition of the Schools." *Chicago Tribune*. April 5, 1865. newspapers.com/image/349382861.

Bolker, Norman, MD. "Doctors on Horseback: The Practice of Medicine in Washington Territory." *Medical Bulletin.* Fall 1989: 20+.

Bond, Rowland. "The Ruins' Red Glare Disclosed No Despair." *Spokane Daily Chronicle.* August 5, 1964: 3+.

"Books Wanted at Poor Farm: A Single Story of Adventure Was Re-Read and Discussed." March 13, 1896. newspapers.com/image/565982619.

Bragg, L. E. *More than Petticoats: Remarkable Washington Women.* Guilford, CT: TwoDot / Morris Book Publishing, LLC, 1998.

"Brewery Claims Customer: Says Dr. Latham, Dry Adherent, Purchased Much Beer." *Semi-Weekly Spokesman-Review.* October 31, 1914. newspapers.com/image/56652656.

Brooklyn Daily Eagle. April 16, 1893 (New York) 4.

"Builders and Leaders: Mary A. Latham." *Spokesman-Review.* May 27, 2007. newspapers.com/image/577037532.

"Builders and Leaders: The *Spokesman-Review* Bronzes." spokesman.com/about/builders-and-leaders/.

"Burnt District: Diagram of the Blocks Swept Over by the Flames." *Spokane Chronicle.* August 4, 1989. newspapers.com/image/566571451.

"Butte Woman Seeks Property—Latham Will Case—Alleged Hiding of Document." *Butte Daily Post.* August 13, 1904. newspapers.com/image/348769277.

"Called to Alaska." *Spokane Chronicle.* April 2, 1898. newspapers.com/image/562172151.

Cemetery Record: James Latham. Greenwood Memorial Terrace, Office of Secretary of State, Washington State Archives, Digital Archives, digitalarchives.wa.gov.

Chicago Tribune. September 2, 1893, (Illinois) 6.

———. November 2, 1893, (Illinois) 7.

Cochran, Barbara F. *Seven Frontier Women and the Founding of Spokane Falls.* Spokane, WA: Tornado Creek Publications, 2011.

"Coming Home: Dr. Latham Doesn't Think the Alaska Country Is Just a Paradise." *Spokane Chronicle.* July 22, 1898. newspapers.com/image/562174479.

"Complete Lecture: Full Report of the Paper Read by Dr. Carey at the Biochemic Convention." *Spokane Chronicle.* May 30, 1891. newspapers.com/image/562160708.

Conner, Eliza Archard. *"E. A." Abroad: A Summer in Europe.* Cincinnati, OH: W. E. Dibble & Co. (1883).

———. "Woman's World in Paragraphs: How Two Splendid Girls Made a Home for Themselves." *Crawford County Forum.* (1890, December 19). newspapers.com/image/600969689.

———. "Woman's World in Paragraphs: A Woman Farmer's Southdown Sheep and Jersey Cows." *Monmouth Press.* (Atlantic Highlands, NJ) (1893, July 15). newspapers.com/image/375970157.

———. "A Woman in Alaska: Eliza Archard Conner Writes of the Yukon River Route." *Harrisburg Telegraph.* (1898, September 27). newspapers.com/image/44274574.

———. "Susan B. Anthony." *Evening Statesman* (Walla Walla, WA). (1907, March 8). newspapers.com/image/194807691.

"County Will Build Home for Poor Consumptives: Plan 20 Room House at the County Poor Farm near Spangle." *Spokane Chronicle.* June 26, 1907. newspapers.com/image/561624881.

"Courthouse History." spokanecounty.org/2243/Courthouse-History.

Culver, Nina. "Sorosis Club a Spokane Institution for 105 Years." *Spokesman-Review.* January 28, 1996. spokesman.com/stories/1996/jan/28sorosis-club-a-spokane-institution-for-105-years/.

Day, Mary Edith. "A Line of Strong Women." *Our Mountain Home* (Talladega, AL). April 16, 1902. newspapers.com/image/306641192.

"Deserted and Destitute: The Mother Was Sick and the Children Crying for Bread." *Spokane Review.* October 26, 1892. newspapers.com/image/565971239.

"Died of a Broken Heart: Is Said Chief Joseph's Death Was Due to His Grief and Worry." *Evening Statesman* (Walla Walla, WA). September 29, 1904. newspapers.com/image/148726426.

"Directory of the City of Spokane Falls for the Year 1887." Compiled by Charles E. Reeves. Spokane Falls, Washington Territory: Spokane Printing Co., 1887.

"Doctor Delighted, and Writes an Enthusiastic Letter Back East." *Spokane Falls Review.* June 2, 1889. newspapers.com/image/565844778.

"Doctors Fell Out: They Were Husband and Wife, and Are Separated." *Cincinnati Enquirer.* July 26, 1895. newspapers.com/image/32567989.

"Dr. E. H. Latham, Pioneer, Dies: Came to Spokane in 1888—Practiced Medicine on Okanogan Reservation 29 Years." *Semi-Weekly Spokesman-Review.* May 29, 1928. newspapers.com/image/567164185.

"Dr. George Conner Dead." *Cincinnati Enquirer.* January 14, 1897. newspapers.com/image/34467293.

"Dr. Latham a Fugitive: Driving Across Country from Her Home at Mead with Officer in Hot Pursuit—New Warrant Issued." *Spokane Chronicle.* July 25, 1905. newspapers.com/image/562323604.

"Dr. Latham a Prisoner: Declared She Was Out on a Camping Trip with Friends." *Evening Statesman* (Walla Walla, WA). August 2, 1905. newspapers.com/image/149457944.

"Dr. Latham Has Gone." *Spokane Chronicle.* June 16, 1898. newspapers.com/image/562173720.

"Dr. Latham Is a Winner: She Can Keep Her Homestead Says Register Ludden." *Spokane Chronicle.* August 5, 1899. newspapers.com/image/562115843.

"Dr. Latham Is in Serious Plight: The Evidence Piles Up Against Her in Trial for Arson." *Spokane Review.* June 14, 1905. Retrieved from historical files of Northwest Room at Spokane Public Library, Main Branch.

"Dr. Latham Is Starving: Could Not Appear in Court to Receive Sentence." *Spokesman-Review.* July 2, 1905. Retrieved from historical files of Northwest Room at Spokane Public Library, Main Branch.

"Dr. Latham Puts Up a Fight: In Effort to Get Out of Prison, Makes Startling Allegations." *Evening Statesman* (Walla Walla, WA). July 23, 1906. newspapers.com/image/201704294.

"Dr. Latham Recaptured: Found Stranded and Alone in Hoodoo Valley." *Rathdrum Tribune.* August 4, 1905. newspapers.com/image/605133963.

"Dr. Latham Sued Again: The Spokane Drug Company Wants Pay for Goods." *Spokane Chronicle.* August 5, 1905. newspapers.com/image/562033252.

"Dr. Latham Sues Prall: Says Her Former Friend Is Still Owing Her Money." *Spokane Chronicle.* May 7, 1908. newspapers.com/image/562358980.

"Dr. Latham Was Granger." *Semi-Weekly Spokesman-Review.* November 24, 1912. newspapers.com/image/566188124.

"Dr. Latham's Latest Boast." *Spokane Press.* August 19, 1904. newspapers.com/image/149358271.

"Dr. Latham's Memory Was Again in Trouble." *Spokane Press.* October 21, 1905. newspapers.com/image/87712750.

"Dr. Latham's View of It." *Spokane Chronicle.* January 16, 1894. newspapers.com/image/565841112.

"Dr. Latham's Voyage: She Says Alaska Is a Wonderful Place." *Spokane Chronicle.* July 7, 1898. newspapers.com/image/562174162.

"Dr. Mary A. Latham Dead; Came to Spokane in 1888—Falls Victim to Pneumonia and Passes Away at Sacred Heart Hospital." *Spokane Chronicle.* January 20, 1917. newspapers.com/image/563571548.

"Dr. Mary A. Latham Dies: Pioneer Woman Physician Succumbs to Pneumonia." *Semi-Weekly Spokesman-Review.* January 21, 1917. newspapers.com/image/566609483.

"Dr. Mary Latham Again Behind Bars: Noted Woman Ex-Convict Faces Criminal Practice Charge." *Semi-Weekly Spokesman-Review.* July 7, 1908. newspapers.com/image/566451013.

"Dr. Mary Latham Case Is Dismissed." *Spokane Chronicle.* November 11, 1911. newspapers.com/image/562160020.

"Dr. Mary Latham Comes Home Again—and Tells a Seattle Reporter How to Carry His Dresses." *Spokane Chronicle.* October 24, 1898. newspapers.com/image/562104117.

"Dr. Mary Latham Estate Is $3,000: Pioneer Leaves No Will—Son Asks Letters of Administration." *Spokane Chronicle.* February 1, 1917. newspapers.com/image/563578453.

"Dr. Mary Latham Goes to Panama." *Spokane Chronicle.* November 14, 1911. newspapers.com/image/562160097.

"Dr. Mary Latham Got Bewildered in Idaho Woods and Was Caught." *Spokane Press.* August 1, 1905. newspapers.com/image/149321834.

"Dr. Mary Latham Is Found Guilty: Jury Reaches a Verdict in about Two Hours." June 1905. *Biography N.W.* Retrieved from historical files of Northwest Room at Spokane Public Library, Main Branch.

"Dr. Mary Sued by Attorney." *Spokane Press.* January 4, 1905. newspapers.com/image/149217994.

"Dr. Mary Sued by Lawyers." *Spokane Press.* July 28, 1905. chroniclingamerica.loc.gov/lccn/sn88085947/1905-07-28/ed-1/

"Dr. W. F. Lamson Weds." *Kennewick Courier.* July 30, 1909. newspapers.com/image/70957411.

"Dress Reformers Day: Chief Topic of Discussion in Women's Congress at Fair." *Seattle Post-Intelligencer.* May 17, 1893. newspapers.com/image/332929665.

"Editorials by Women." *Semi-Weekly Spokesman-Review.* March 13, 1900. newspapers.com/image/566007432.

"Editors Have Troubles Too: Wood Gets a Half Interest in the *Stevens County Reveille*." *Spokane Chronicle.* March 8, 1902. newspapers.com/image/561641187.

Edwards, Rev. Jonathan. *An Illustrated History of Spokane County, State of Washington.* San Francisco: W. H. Lever, 1900.

Evening Telegraph. October 25, 1893 (Ohio) 2.

"Exit the Poor Farm, Here Since 1888: Indigent Care Started with Rare $2.50." *Spokesman Review.* July 15, 1945. Retrieved from historical files of Northwest Room at Spokane Public Library, Main Branch.

"Father's Alleged Cruelty." *Spokesman-Review.* April 23, 1903. newspapers.com/image/565587389.

"Firebrand." *Spokesman-Review.* January 12, 1983. newspapers.com/image/571971058.

"First White Child Born in New Richmond Died Thursday of Last Week." Copied by Warren Latham, North 1017 Washington Street, Spokane, Washington, August 1934. (Original clipping in possession of Mrs. J. W. [Mary] Scribner, Route #1, Chattaroy, Washington.) Courtesy of Glenn M. Latham Collection. January 26, 2019.

"Flower Seeds to Give Away." *Spokane Chronicle*. March 17, 1900. newspapers.com/image/562172360.

"For a Good Cause: Mrs. Latham Pitches into People Who Are 'Stuck Up' on Account of Wealth." *Spokane Review*. June 4, 1891. newspapers.com/image/566003818.

"For Sweet Charity's Sake: Newsboys and Bootblacks Will Dine Free New Year's Night." *Spokane Falls Review*. December 30, 1890. newspapers.com/image/565842140.

"For the Relief Fund: World's Fair Receipts Next Sunday to Go to the Firemen." *Chicago Tribune*. July 13, 1893. newspapers.com/image/349831442.

"Formally Opened: The New Home for the Friendless Formally Dedicated Yesterday Afternoon." *Spokane Falls Review*. May 23, 1890. newspapers.com/image/565849709.

"Former Friend Hurts Dr. Latham: Nellie Standsbury Tells Hard Story of Arson at Mead." *Semi-Weekly Spokesman-Review*. June 13, 1905. Retrieved from historical files of Northwest Room at Spokane Public Library, Main Branch.

"Fortune Waits for Little Girl Sought in the Inland Empire." *Spokane Chronicle*. December 25, 1915. newspapers.com/image/562198612.

"Found Her Real Jennie: Dr. Latham Says She Has Located the Missing Woman." *Spokane Chronicle*. September 10, 1904. newspapers.com/image/562047397.

"Four Plead Not Guilty: Fenn Says He Didn't Assault Dr. Mary Latham." *Spokane Chronicle*. June 17, 1899. newspapers.com/image/562115505.

"Four Years for Dr. Mary Latham." *Spokane Chronicle*. July 20, 1905. newspapers.com/image/562322006.

"Fruit Men Organize—Meet at the City Hall and Form a New Society." *Spokane Chronicle*. February 3, 1900. newspapers.com/image/562170966.

Gidley, Mick. *With One Sky Above Us: Life on An Indian Reservation at the Turn of the Century*. New York: G. P. Putman's Sons, 1979.

"Give the Doctors Justice." *Spokane Chronicle*. September 5, 1903. newspapers.com/image/561602450.

"Go Back! Go Back!—That's the Cry of the Gold Hunters on the Yukon." *Spokane Chronicle.* August 29, 1898. newspapers.com/image/562175050.

"Hard Luck Tales Given Deaf Ear: Dr. M. A. Latham Declares She Is Through with Most Charity Work Now." *Spokane Chronicle.* April 5, 1911. newspapers.com/image/562174379.

"Has Mary Latham Skipped Country?" *Spokane Press.* July 25, 1905. newspapers.com/image/149319447.

Hawthorne, Julian. *History of Washington: The Evergreen State from Early Dawn to Daylight, Volume 2.* New York: American Historical Publications, 1893.

"Heap Bad Cold: Indians Dying from La Grippe on the Colville Reservation." *Butte Weekly Miner.* April 16, 1891. newspapers.com/image/348979356.

Hengen, Nona. *In Pursuit of Compassion: A Centennial History of the Spokane Humane Society, 1897–1997.* Spokane, WA: Spokane Humane Society, 1997.

"History of Medicine Timeline." datesandevents.org/events-timelines/10-history-of-medicine-timeline.html.

"History of the Parker Family and Academy." parkeracademy-nsfreu.weebly.com

Hoffman, Peter B., PhD. *History of the Federal Parole System.* May 2003, 7. justice.gov/sites/default/files/uspc/legacy/2009/10/07/history.pdf.

"Homestead Act of 1862." https://www.nps.gov/articles/the-homestead-act.htm.

"Hospital for Women." *Spokane Review.* October 22, 1891. newspapers.com/image/565844847.

"Hospital for Women: It Will Be Built on the Corner of Post and Main Streets." *Spokane Review.* December 6, 1891. newspapers.com/image/565846301.

"Hospitals." *Spokane Chronicle.* April 13, 1905. newspapers.com/image/561552809.

"Humane Society at Work: Membership Strengthened by Names of Prominent Citizens." *Semi-Weekly Spokesman-Review.* June 3, 1896. newspapers.com/image/565983588.

Hunt, Linda Lawrence. *Bold Spirit: Helga Estby's Forgotten Walk Across Victorian America*. New York: Anchor Books, 2005.

Hyslop, Robert B. "The Spokane Fire." *Spokane's Building Blocks*. Spokane, WA: R. B. Hyslop, 1983.

"I Didn't Do It, That's All: We Had Bitter Enemies—Dr. Latham Says that They Threatened to Burn Out Her Store." *Spokane Chronicle*. July 11, 1905. newspapers.com/image/562319237.

"Inspected the Hospital." *Spokane Chronicle*. February 6, 1897. newspapers.com/image/562028830.

"Internal Revenue Service (IRS) Historical Study: IRS Historical Fact Book: A Chronology 1646-1992." governmentattic.org/5docs/IRS-HistoricalFactBook_1992.pdf.

"In the Cause of Charity." *Semi-Weekly Spokesman-Review*. March 8, 1894. newspapers.com/image/565832293.

"In the Superior Court." *Semi-Weekly Spokesman-Review*. October 24, 1916. newspapers.com/image/566521494.

"In Violation of the City Ordinance: Disreputable Places Running on Sunday as Well as on Other Days." *Spokane Chronicle*. September 26, 1902. newspapers.com/image/562038786.

"Is Direct from Dawson: News Brought by the Steamer *New England*." *Semi-Weekly Spokesman-Review*. July 6, 1898. newspapers.com/image/566385393.

"Is Dr. Latham the Conspirator? Defense Tries to Prove That, Jilted by Dr. Messner, She Plans His Ruin—In Fine Form, Convicted Arsonist Tells of Betrayal." *Semi-Weekly Spokesman-Review*. October 24, 1905. newspapers.com/image/566039963.

"Is Dr. Latham Trifling with Court?" *Spokane Press*. August 16, 1904. newspapers.com/image/149357341.

"It Is Put Off: The Chase Trial Postponed for Ten Days Until Prosecutor Fenton Returns." *Spokane Chronicle*. January 15, 1894. newspapers.com/image/565841043.

Jackson, J. C. "The Work of the Anti-Saloon League." *The Annals of the American Academy of Political and Social Science*, vol. 32, *Regulation of the Liquor Traffic* (November 1908), 12–26.

Jones, Arthur. "Great Hustlers: A Neat Compliment to Spokaneites [*sic*] and Their Enterprise." *Spokesman-Review*. January 17, 1889. newspapers.com/image/566439675.

"Journeymen Plumbers." *Spokane Chronicle*. March 12, 1898. newspapers.com/image/562171379.

"Judge Questions Dr. Mary Latham." *Semi-Weekly Spokesman-Review*. November 18, 1916. newspapers.com/image/566614428.

"Jury to Try Dr. Latham: Prosecuting Attorney Barnhart Dispenses with Examination." *Semi-Weekly Spokesman-Review*. May 18, 1905. newspapers.com/image/566293886.

Kershner, Jim. "Jim Kershner's 100 Years Ago Today." *Spokesman-Review*. May 20, 2020.

"King of Klondike: 'Big Alec' MacDonald and How He Got His Millions." *Marion Star*. September 9, 1898. newspapers.com/image/299555851.

"Klondike Craze: A Syndicate of Women Are Arranging to Go Next Spring." *Spokane Chronicle*. August 23, 1897. newspapers.com/image/562117568.

"Klondike Missionaries: Interesting Letter Recounting the Experiences of Two Ministers." *Akron Beacon Journal*. January 27, 1898. newspapers.com/image/228054887.

"Labor Day in Spokane: Men of Brains and Brawn Are Having a Royal Holiday." *Spokane Chronicle*. September 5, 1898. newspapers.com/image/562103295.

Lamberson, Carolyn. "Best and Brightest: Spokane-Area Women, Past and Present, Blaze Trails." *Spokesman-Review*. November 13, 2019. Section: "serendipity."

Latham, Mary A. Letter to the editor, *Spokane Falls Review* (1890a, December 23). newspapers.com/image/565841331.

———. "The Queer Mascot." *Spokane Falls Review* (1890b, December 25). newspapers.com/image/565841585.

———. "Women as Physicians: Mrs. Mary A. Latham, of Spokane, Ably Discusses the Matter." *Spokane Chronicle* (1891a, January 23). newspapers.com/image/562158917.

———. Letter to the editor, *Semi-Weekly Spokesman-Review* (1891b, February 5). newspapers.com/image/565831042.

———. Letter to the editor, *Spokane Falls Review* (1891c, March 17). newspapers.com/image/566018282.

———. "Stories of Canines." *Spokane Review* (1891d, July 2). newspapers.com/image/565835559.

———. Letter to the editor, *Spokane Chronicle* (1891e, July 2). newspapers.com/image/562929556.

———. Letter to the editor, *Spokane Chronicle* (1891f, August 11). newspapers.com/image/562930193.

———. "The Love of Money: A Very Good Sermon Written by a Woman." *Spokane Review* (1891g, August 16). newspapers.com/image/565837364.

———. Letter to the editor, *Spokane Review* (1892a, June 5). newspapers.com/image/565967448.

———. "Christian Science: Its Fallacies and Absurdities as They Appear to Dr. Latham." *Spokane Review* (1892b, September 17). newspapers.com/image/565960045.

———. Letter to the editor, *Spokane Chronicle* (1895, July 23). newspapers.com/image/561481293.

———. Letter to the editor, *Spokane Chronicle* (1897, December 21). newspapers.com/image/562127293.

———. Letter to the editor, *Spokane Chronicle* (1898a, January 29). newspapers.com/image/562116734.

———. Letter to the editor, *Spokane Chronicle* (1898b, December 14). newspapers.com/image/562105275.

———. Letter to the editor, *Semi-Weekly Spokesman-Review* (1899, March 12). newspapers.com/image/566379223.

———. Letter to the editor, *Spokane Chronicle* (1901a, January 17). newspapers.com/image/562111403.

———. Letter to the editor, *Semi-Weekly Spokesman-Review* (1901b, February 25). newspapers.com/image/566358230.

———. Letter to the editor, *Spokane Chronicle* (1902a, June 11). newspapers.com/image/562033952.

———. Letter to the editor, *Semi-Weekly Spokesman-Review* (1902b, October 9). newspapers.com/image/566358970.

———. Letter to the editor, *Spokane Chronicle* (1902c, October 9). newspapers.com/image/562039423.

Latham, Warren. "Three Years' Work Among the Poor: Warren Latham and His Wife Are Obliged to Leave Spokane." *Spokane Chronicle*. December 8, 1899. newspapers.com/image/561488768.

"Line of Strong Women." *Our Mountain Home*. April 16, 1902. newspapers.com/image/306641192.

"Lionberger/Witcraft Family Tree." *Ancestry.com*. ancestry.com/familytree/tree/78310768/family.

"Little Girl Was Lost." *Spokane Chronicle*. May 1, 1901. newspapers.com/image/562114414.

"Lodging: Rooms $200 a Month at Dawson City." *Dayton Herald*. September 28, 1898. newspapers.com/image/392155581.

"Loved Her Too Well: D. W. Hoskins Murders Ida Bennett and Suicides." *Spokane Review*. May 6, 1893. newspapers.com/image/565989075.

"Lying on a Stretcher, Dr. Mary Latham Receives Her Sentence: Hauled to Court House in Ambulance." *Spokane Press*. July 20, 1905. newspapers.com/image/149317863.

Mansky, Jacqueline. "The Medical Practitioner Who Paved the Way for Women Doctors in America." smithsonianmag.com/science-nature/woman-who-paved-way-female-physicians-america-180967104/.

"Mary A. Latham's Homestead: She Asks for a Year's Leave of Absence." *Semi-Weekly Spokesman-Review*. June 2, 1898. newspapers.com/image/566383456.

"Mary Latham Is Arrested for Burning Her Drug Store—Prosecuting Attorney [*sic*] Believe They Have Good Case Against Mary Stanbury, Woman Who is Thought to Have Obeyed Dr. Latham's Orders and Burned Drug Store." *Spokane Press*. May 10, 1905. newspapers.com/image/149277527.

"Mary Latham Taken to the Penitentiary: Aged Physician Leaves the County Jail in Company with Thieves, Hold-Up Men and Other

Dangerous Criminals." *Spokane Press*. January 9, 1906. newspapers
.com/image/194686788.

"Matron Appointed." *Evening Statesman* (Walla Walla, WA). November
8, 1905. newspapers.com/image/149489491.

"Medical Congress: Pan-American Gathering in the City of Mexico." *Spokesman Review*. November 19, 1896. newspapers.com/
image/566353717.

"Messner and Prall Sought Latham's Money to Appeal Her Case." *Spokane Press*. October 24, 1905. newspapers.com/image/149356533.

"Messner Woos as Shop Burns: He Visits Widow While Store at
Mead Is Blazing." *Semi-Weekly Spokesman-Review*. June 17, 1905.
Retrieved from historical files of Northwest Room at Spokane Pub-
lic Library, Main Branch.

"Miles Poindexter Papers, 1897–1940." archiveswest.orbiscascade.org/
ark:/80444/xv57473.

"Millions Lost: An Appalling Calamity Visits the Proud City of Spokane Falls." *Spokane Chronicle*. August 5, 1989. newspapers.com/
image/566571451.

"Miss Neilson Will Not Submit: The Work of the Commission of Physicians Amounts to But Little." *Spokane Review*. January 15, 1894.
newspapers.com/image/565969842.

Monmouth Press. July 15, 1893 (New Jersey) 7.

"More Prizes for Babies: Two Years Will Be the Age Limit for the
Little Folks." *Spokane Chronicle*. October 13, 1899. newspapers.com/
image/561487922.

"More than a World's Fair." *Evening Telegraph* (Bucyrus, OH). October
25, 1893. newspapers.com/image/600593582.

"Mrs. Latham Confesses." *Spokane Press*. August 23, 1905. newspapers
.com/image/149330303.

"Mrs. Latham's Protégé: Has Found a Home with John Crabb's
Family." *Spokane Review*. January 6, 1893. newspapers.com/
image/565973151.

"Mrs. Latham Wants Bed." *Spokane Press*. August 15, 1904. newspapers
.com/image/149356917.

"Must Show the Papers: Dr. Latham Is Ordered to Produce Power of Attorney." *Spokane Chronicle.* August 23, 1904. newspapers.com/image/562046971.

"Mystery of Illness of Rose Elliott Solved: Girl Pays Penalty of Acts—Criminal Operation Was Performed." *Spokane Press.* April 24, 1901. newspapers.com/image/150494545.

National Science Foundation (NSF) under Grant #1659467 to W. J. Landon and S. Jones. n.d. "Parker Academy: A Place for Freedom, a Space for Resistance." parkeracademy-nsfreu.weebly.com.

"New Librarian Chosen: A Deadlock in the Commission—Frank Price Elected." *Spokane Review.* January 9, 1894. newspapers.com/image/565969016.

"New School Board: Directors of the Library Association Want Mrs. Latham." *Spokane Review.* November 3, 1891. newspapers.com/image/565843306.

"Newspaper Woman Weds." *Spokesman-Review.* March 13, 1913. newspapers.com/image/566524025.

"No Bail for Dr. Latham: Woman Accused of Arson Has Not Gotten Bondsmen Yet." *Semi-Weekly Spokesman-Review.* May 13, 1905. newspapers.com/image/566291405.

"No Room for a Clubhouse." *Spokane Weekly Review.* March 3, 1892. newspapers.com/image/565832540.

"Northwest Aids Building Record: Spokane and Other Western Cities Prepare for Opening of Panama Canal." *Spokane Chronicle.* February 13, 1912. newspapers.com/image/562141213.

"Obituary: Dr. George Conner." ancestry.com/mediaui-viewer/tree/78310768/person/400127320991/media/e60f15d2-23ed-4b57-a903-52e84eefb825?usePUBJs=true

"Occupational Licenses, Registers, and Directories." Ancestry.com. ancestry.com/interactive/9207/42859_2221301551_2573-00350?pid=602933&backurl=https://www.ancestry.com/family-tree/person/tree/78310768/.

"On an Old Duebill: Suit for a Block of Le Roi Mining Stock—Mrs. Mary Latham Demands That Col. Ridpath Shall Deliver It or Pay the Value." *Semi-Weekly Spokesman-Review.* March 3, 1897. newspapers.com/image/566377814.

"Orchard in Dispute." *Semi-Weekly Spokesman-Review*. January 19, 1895. newspapers.com/image/566351268.

Otgaar, Henry, Peter Muris, Mark L. Howe, and Harald Merckelbach. "What Drives False Memories in Psychopathy?" *SAGE Clinical Psychological Science*. ncbi.nlm.nih.gov/pmc/articles/PMC5665161/.

"Our New York Letter: The Rush to the Klondike Is Assuming Notable Proportions." *Akron Beacon Journal*. February 4, 1898. newspapers .com/image/228054936.

"Over the Hills to the Poor House." *Spokesman-Review*. August 29, 1915. newspapers.com/image/566606059.

"Pardon Denied Doctor Mary Latham." *Spokane Press*. July 24, 1906. newspapers.com/image/194746007.

"Pardoned for Crime She Never Committed: Dr. Mary A. Latham Offers Reward for Conviction of Arson." *Spokane Chronicle*. February 28, 1908. newspapers.com/image/561734263.

"Paris and Her Show: Eliza Archard Conner on the Great Exposition." *Kenosha Evening News*. April 4, 1900. newspapers.com/image/595101783.

Parker, Sarah Preston Baker. n.d. "A Brief History of Clermont Academy, Together with a Few Items from the Lives of Its Founder & Principal." Courtesy of Greg Roberts Collection.

"Pays $10,000 for 160-Acre Farm: Dr. Mary Latham to Have Sanitorium at Long Lake." *Semi-Weekly Spokesman-Review*. October 20, 1912. newspapers.com/image/566176524.

Pence, Lawrence, MD. "A Very Brief History of the Spokane County Medical Society." *Medical Bulletin*. Fall 1989: 9.

"Pen, Chisel and Brush." *Atchison Daily Globe*. April 22, 1893. newspapers.com/image/479972735.

"People's Voice: A Woman's Reason—Why She Voted Against Mrs. Mary Latham." *Spokane Review*. November 10, 1891. newspapers .com/image/565844004.

"Philippine-American War: Filipino History." *Encyclopedia Britannica*. britannica.com/event/Philippine-American-War.

"Plucky Woman War Correspondent: Eliza Archard Conner, Who is Carrying a Typewriter Around the World." *Fort Wayne Sentinel*.

June 24, 1899. ancestry.com/interactive /6178/news-fortwayne-fws entenel.1899_06_24_0011?pid=471556107&backurl=https://www .ancestry.com/family-tree/.

"Plumbers Deplore Latham's Death." *Spokane Press*. April 22, 1903. newspapers.com/image/149348867.

"Polk & Co., R. L., Spokane City Directory, 1890, 1892–93, and 1896." Washington State Archives, Digital Archives, digitalarchives.wa.gov.

"Poor Farm Investigation: Members of the Ladies' Benevolent Society Will Attend at Spangle." *Spokane Review*. June 10, 1892. newspapers.com/image/565968430.

"Prison Commission Has Additional Findings and Figures for Governor." *Evening Statesman* (Walla Walla, WA). January 1, 1907. newspapers.com/image/194783572.

"Pullman: Professor Searches for Truth about Old Prisons." *Kitsap Sun*. products.kitsapsun.com/archive/1995/01-02/303538_pullman_professor_searches_for.html.

Ranch and Range (Yakima, WA). February 15, 1900. newspapers.com/ image/88273274.

"Rare Curios from the North: Dr. Mary A. Latham Has Received a Fine Collection." *Spokane Chronicle*. October 3, 1901. newspapers .com/image/562108910.

Rathdrum Tribune. (Rathdrum, ID) Various issues.

"Re-elected Baldwin: Library Association Selects Officers—Lee Fairchild's Lecture." *Spokane Review*. January 3, 1893. newspapers.com/ image/565972026.

"Richard M. Barnhart 1869–1910." Posted by Merliene Andre Bendixen. September 10, 2010. iagenweb.org/boards/emmet/obituaries/ index.cgi?read=297663.

Rockey, J. L. *History of Clermont County, Ohio, with Illustrations and Biographical Sketches of Its Prominent Men and Pioneers*. Philadelphia: Press of J. B. Lippincott & Co., 1880.

"Royalty Figures in Latham Will: Dr. Latham Said Jennie 'C.' Johnson was a Member of Swedish Aristocracy." *Semi-Weekly Spokesman-Review*. August 13, 1904. newspapers.com/image/566019486.

Russell, Julie Y. "Sisters of St. Francis, Fairmount Cemetery." *Spokane Historical.* spokanehistorical.org/items/show/138.

Russell, Julie Y. "Spokane's Deadliest Disaster, Greenwood Cemetery." *Spokane Historical.* spokanehistorical.org/items/show/136.

"Sad, Sad Story: How a Happy Family Was Broken Up by a Designing Fiend." *Spokane Chronicle.* October 2, 1891. newspapers.com/image/562931440.

"Salvation Army: A Writer Who Votes the Organization a Nuisance." *Spokane Review.* February 24, 1892. newspapers.com/image/565987538.

San Juan Islander. March 9, 1907 (Washington) 2.

"Says Her Dead Son Comes Back Each Night." *Spokane Chronicle.* June 22, 1905. newspapers.com/image/562310920.

"Say the Trees Were N. G." *Spokane Chronicle.* April 9, 1895. newspapers.com/image/562071204.

"Scattering Klondike Gold: How Swiftwater Bill Remembered a Spokane Friend." *Spokane Chronicle.* March 24, 1898. newspapers.com/image/562171889.

Schlicke, Carl P., MD. "Spokane, A Community of Hospitals." *Medical Bulletin.* Fall 1989: 31.

"School Board: The Name is Advanced of Mrs. Mary A. Latham." *Spokane Review.* November 1, 1891. newspapers.com/image/565843133.

Schultz, R. A. "Alexander F. MacLeod House." *Spokane Historical.* spokanehistorical.org/items/show/599.

Seattle Post-Intelligencer. Various issues.

———. May 17, 1893 (Washington) 1.

"Second Serious Mishap at Paris Exposition: Panic on a Bridge Causes the Death of Two and Injuring of Many Persons." *Seattle Post-Intelligencer.* August 19, 1900. newspapers.com/image/333661093.

Semi-Weekly Spokesman-Review. Various issues.

"Sentence at This Time Might Kill Doctor Latham." *Spokane Chronicle.* July 19, 1905. newspapers.com/image/562321729.

"Set Adrift in the City: Without a Friend to Help Her in a Time of Trouble." *Spokane Chronicle.* January 5, 1900. newspapers.com/image/562169672.

"She Cut a Needle Out of Her: Dr. Mary Latham Performs a Delicate Operation." *Semi-Weekly Spokesman-Review.* February 19, 1898. newspapers.com/image/566377494.

"She Is a Deputy Sheriff." *Spokane Chronicle.* April 18, 1896. newspapers.com/image/561483773.

"She Keeps Her Ranch: The Noted Contest for Dr. Latham's Land is Ended." *Spokane Chronicle.* March 27, 1901. newspapers.com/image/562113736.

"Sheriff Probes the Latham Fire: Mead Conflagration Causes Investigation of Its Cause to Be Set Afoot." *Semi-Weekly Spokesman-Review.* May 9, 1905. newspapers.com/image/566289830.

"She Terrified the Neighbors: Mrs. William E. Stevenson Goes Insane and Flourishes a Revolver." *Semi-Weekly Spokesman-Review.* March 7, 1897. newspapers.com/image/566377913.

"Sickening Story." *Spokane Review.* October 7, 1892. newspapers.com/image/565965813.

"Smallpox Among the Indians: Thirty Cases, and Spreading Among the Nespelins [*sic*]." January 28, 1900. newspapers.com/image/333585124.

Spokane Chronicle. Various issues.

Spokane Falls Review. Various issues.

"Spokane Men in Dawson: Gus. Seiffert Is There—George Foster, Col. O. V. Davis, Swiftwater Bill and Many More." *Spokane Chronicle.* September 17, 1898. newspapers.com/image/562103435.

Spokane Police Department History Book Committee. *Life Behind the Badge, Volume II: The Spokane Police Department's Turbulent Years, 1903–1923.* Marceline, MO: Walsworth Publishing and Printing Company, 2010.

Spokane Press. Various issues.

Spokane Review. Various issues.

"Spokane Route to the Klondike: Cyrene, the Celebrated Dancer, Who Is Now in the City, Writes a Pretty Ballad." *Spokane Chronicle.* March 5, 1898. newspapers.com/image/562171142.

Spokesman-Review. Various issues.

———. "Monument Honors Doctor Who Was Community Pioneer: Mary Latham Treated Women, Children and Poor." April 5, 2007. newspapers.com/image/576998681.

"Start a New Magazine." *Spokane Chronicle*. March 19, 1901. newspapers.com/image/562113462.

State of Washington: In the matter of the estate of James Latham, deceased, Case No. 3068, various documents (Superior Court, Spokane County, 1904).

State of Washington: *Jennie H. Johnson vs. Mary A. Latham and John H. Mesner* [sic], Case No. 19384, various documents (Superior Court, Spokane County, 1904).

State of Washington vs. Bertha Wardrum, Case No. 1-1448, various documents (Superior Court, Spokane County, 1905).

State of Washington vs. Mary A. Latham, Case No. 1-2438, various documents (Superior Court, Spokane County, 1905).

"State Teachers' Association." *Daily Empire*. July 7, 1859. newspapers.com/image/79841433.

"Stories of Street and Town." *Lewiston Inter-State News*. August 11, 1905. newspapers.com/image/375426857.

"Swiftwater Kept His Word: Dr. Latham Says She Can Build Her Hospital at Dawson Any Time She Chooses." *Spokane Chronicle*. October 28, 1898. newspapers.com/image/562104224.

"Terrible Cruelty: Unfortunate Kitty Darragh's Experience." *Spokane Daily Chronicle*. July 8, 1890. newspapers.com/image/562144219.

"This Is the Babies' Day: Little Folks of Spokane Compete for Honors." *Spokane Chronicle*. October 16, 1899. newspapers.com/image/561487955.

"This Is the County Poor Farm." *Spokesman-Review*. November 22, 1903. newspapers.com/image/566015060.

"Three Thousand: Cases of Typhoid Fever in the Metropolis of the Klondike." *Cincinnati Enquirer*. September 27, 1898. newspapers.com/image/32430311.

Tinsley, Jesse. "Then and Now: Eastern State Hospital." *Spokesman-Review*. July 4, 2016. newspapers.com/image/581673804.

"Too Many Wanted It: Earnest's Bail Bond Is in Lively Demand." *Spokane Chronicle*. December 12, 1901. newspapers.com/image/561635242.

"To Organize a Humane Society: A Number of Ladies and Gentlemen Met Last Night for That Purpose." *Semi-Weekly Spokesman-Review*. May 17, 1896. newspapers.com/image/566376663.

"Trees of Idaho: Idaho Hosts More than 20 Tree Species." Accessed February 27, 2021. idahoforests.org/content-item/trees-of-idaho/.

Twice-Weekly Spokesman-Review. Various issues.

"Two Lucky Little Waifs: Two Sisters Who Are Childless Take Them to Keep." *Semi-Weekly Spokesman-Review*. February 2, 1893. newspapers.com/image/565832232.

"Unclaimed Babe: It Is Found in a Boat at Medical Lake." *Spokane Chronicle*. August 4, 1891. newspapers.com/image/562930073.

"Uncrowned Kings: Dr. Mary Latham Talks on Character to the Good Templars." *Spokane Chronicle*. December 21, 1891. newspapers.com/image/562932828.

"Union Library." *Spokane Review*. April 7, 1892. newspapers.com/image/565989566.

"Union Library Meeting." *Spokane Review*. October 3, 1893. newspapers.com/image/565941062.

US Federal Census Mortality Schedules, 1850–1885. ancestry.com/family-tree/tree/person/tree/78310768/person/400127321118/facts.

US High School Student Lists, 1821–1923. "A Catalogue of the Officers and Students of Phillips Exeter Academy, for the Academical Year 1862–63." ancestry.com/interactive/2395/32216_622204_1295-00004?pid=285949&backurl=https://search.ancestry.com/egi-bin/sse.dll?indiv%3D1%26dbid%3D2.

Valenčius, Conevery Bolton. *The Health of the Country: How American Settlers Understood Themselves and Their Land*. New York: Basic Books, 2002.

"Wanted on Arson Charge." *Lewiston Inter-State News*. August 4, 1905. newspapers.com/image/375426165.

"Warren Latham Says." *Spokesman-Review*. February 10, 1933. newspapers.com/image/567338376.

Washington, County Records 1803–2010. "Spokane, Birth Returns." familysearch.org

———. "Spokane, Death Returns." familysearch.org

"Washington Notes—Spokane." *Kennewick Courier.* March 19, 1909. newspapers.com/image/70954296.

Washington State Archives—Digital Archives. "Corrections Department, Washington State Penitentiary, Commitment Registers and Mug Shots, 1887–1946, Caroline Pearl Richmond, et al." digitalarchives.wa.gov/DigitalObject/Download/43a3e534-c96b-4dde-829c-bcde019e2209.

———. "Corrections Department, Washington State Penitentiary, Commitment Registers and Mug Shots, 1887–1946, Mary Latham." digitalarchives.wa.gov/Record/view/21B0FF061F32086CC90AA86ED0C22?Print-true.

———. "Spokane County Auditor, Death Returns, 1888–1907, Pearl Richmond, H." digitalarchives.wa.gov/Record/View/653203BA1BD9C23A5CAE95B4DF30AA43?Print=true.

"Water Color [*sic*]: A Painting Will Be Voted Away at the Rose Fair." *Spokane Review.* June 11, 1891. newspapers.com/image/566005059.

"What Has the Color of Skin Got to Do with It?" *Santa Cruz Evening News.* August 6, 1909. newspapers.com/image/50560893.

"What Henley Claims." *Spokane Chronicle.* July 21, 1906. newspapers.com/image/561636239.

"Wheat Culture in Washington." *Spokane Chronicle.* January 31, 1894. newspapers.com/image/565841899.

"Who Wants a Child?" *Spokane Chronicle.* September 11, 1899. newspapers.com/image/562116216.

"Who Wants This Baby? Detective McDonald Is Quite Sure He Does Not Need It; Dr. Latham Doesn't." *Spokane Chronicle.* March 10, 1900. newspapers.com/image/562172168.

"Why Two People See the Same Thing But Have Different Memories." *Neuroscience News.com.* neurosciencenews.com/same-event-different-memory-10405.

Wikipedia, s.v. "Dutch Harbor," last modified January 11, 2021, en.wikipedia.org/wiki/Dutch_Harbor.

Wikipedia, s.v. "Exposition Universelle (1900)," last modified January 3, 2021, en.wikipedia.org/wiki/Exposition_Universelle_(1900).

Wikipedia, s.v. "SS *Roanoke,*" last modified December 17, 2020. en.wikipedia.org/wiki/SS_Roanoke.

"Will Dedicate Infirmary April 11." *Spokesman-Review.* April 5, 1914. newspapers.com/image/566496276.

"Witch Wreath at the Museum." hauntedohiobooks.com/news/witch-wreathmuseum/.

"Without a Home: An Infant with Troubles Enough to Be Bald-Headed." *Spokane Review.* December 31, 1892. newspapers.com/image/565984590.

"Women Lawyers Meet." *Fort Scott Daily Monitor.* August 4, 1893. newspapers.com/image/59025886.

"Women Want Panama to Be a Monument of Peace." *Tacoma Times.* February 21, 1912. newspapers.com/image/87712230.

"Worthless Checks Charged to Girl." *Spokane Chronicle.* December 29, 1919. newspapers.com/image/562209147.

Youngs, J. William T. *The Fair and the Falls: Spokane's Expo '74: Transforming an American Environment.* Cheney: Eastern Washington University Press, 1997.

Acknowledgments

Recognition is due to a small army of people who walked with me through unfamiliar territory, until I emerged to find I had written a book—my first.

Thanks to Colorado cousin, Bill Archerd, without whose book, *Archerd: Family History*, I might never have discovered Cousin Mary.

Vicki Latham Watkins and her father, Glenn Marvin Latham, Mary's great-grandson, kindly provided copies of family items, photos, and documents, for which I am very grateful. I hope one day we'll meet.

Thanks for permission to use photographs and other images: Bill Archerd, Erik Highberg, Gary Lewis, and Duane Broyles.

Items mentioned above may not have been included for lack of space, but still, your generosity is greatly appreciated.

Special thanks to Alex Fergus, assistant reference archivist at Joel E. Ferris Research Archives, Northwest Museum of Arts and Culture in Spokane. Working with Alex in the time of coronavirus was a mask-clad pleasure. And to Lee Pierce, archivist at the Eastern Region Branch of the Washington State Archives, thank you for your patience. I should have braved the snowy roads that December day in 2019, but who knew what was about to descend? One day I'll come for that promised tour.

Thanks to the staffs of Washington State Archives—Eastern Region, Olympia Archives, and Office of the Secretary of State, especially Lupita Lopez; University of Washington Libraries—Special Collections; the Ned M. Barnes Northwest Room, Spokane Public Library—particularly librarian Riva Dean for your patience as I piled up books to be reshelved, and for continuing to help after the library closed due to COVID-19; Spokane County Clerk Archives—especially Breanne "Breezy" Hansen; Washington State Department of Corrections, Public Records Unit; City of Spokane Parks and Recreation; Spokane County Auditor's Office; Spokane County Assessor's Office; Spokane City Building Permits Office; and Spokane County Medical Society. Thank you very much, Libby Kamrowski, photographer and newsroom archivist for the

Spokesman-Review; Susan Walker at Spokane Regional Law Enforcement Museum, also Rae Anna Victor; and Jayne Singleton, director of Spokane Valley Heritage Museum, along with volunteer Nancy Pulham. To a person you were encouraging and pleasant.

Thank you, Brian Kobs and Tyson and Julia Voelckers, for helping me understand the world of plat maps and early land records, and for sharing a complete stranger's excitement. Thanks, Kimberly Dailey, for introducing us, and for being a friend.

Heartfelt thanks go across the country to the administrator of the Village of New Richmond, Ohio, Greg Roberts, especially for the personal tour of New Richmond; and to William "Bill" Landon, PhD, Professor of History at Northern Kentucky University, along with Dr. Brian Hackett. Over a period of two years, these three gentlemen generously provided information about the historically relevant Clermont/Parker Academy. Thanks to the Clermont County, Hamilton County, and Ohio Historical Societies. A big thank-you to archivist/curator Gino J. Pasi of the Henry R. Winkler Center for the History of the Health Professions, University of Cincinnati Libraries, for sending me what you imagined was nothing but was really something.

Thank you, Erin Turner, for giving me this opportunity with Globe Pequot/TwoDot. I'll never forget the day—a Friday the 13th—when you wrote, "We want to publish." Thank you for opening the door. Special thanks to Sarah Parke, for taking up where Erin left off, and to Kristen Mellitt for guiding me through the final process to production. Thanks also to Melissa Hayes, one outstanding copyeditor. I feel lucky to have worked with this team of women.

Women Writing the West (WWW) are a support system of inestimable worth. Thank you, Jane Kirkpatrick, for telling me about WWW so long ago in Oregon. The camaraderie and encouragement found at annual conferences—and during recent Zoom meetings—are what give me the courage to continue writing. Good friend and *particeps criminis*, Debra Carey, thanks for always being there.

Love and endless gratitude to my husband, Tom, and to my children, Laura and Brian, for serving as my rally squad and believing in me all these years—that I am a writer, that I could publish a book.